Praise for
Get a Move On!

"I require regular daily exercise to help keep my restless, overactive mind calm; in addition, I use a standing desk and alternate my working body positions with stretching. Luisa not only may well have written the bible for my physical well-being, she has kindly taken the time to write down the why and the how of Mini-Workouts for us all."

—Frederick Marx, author of *Rites to a Good Life: Everyday Rituals of Healing and Transformation* and *At Death Do Us Part* and filmmaker of *Hoop Dreams, Journey from Zanskar,* and *Rites of Passage*

"It is impossible to read this book and not start moving…in the kitchen, at your desk, or anywhere you happen to be. If you're recovering from an injury or looking to ease into exercise but don't know where to start, this book makes it easy and fun with simple exercises, practical tips, and a lot of charm."

—Amy Tucker, game designer

"This is a little book that felt like a big permission slip, freeing me up to feel good about Mini-Workouts. *Get a Move On!* provides a wonderful service for body and spirit."

—Virginia Hume, author of *Haven Point*

"I am absolutely charmed by this book. Herein lies a well-organized, relatable, and informative guide that teaches all of us how to insert healthy bursts of movement into our seemingly mundane routines. I applaud the author's ability to make these tasks meaningful and fun. This is the epitome of progress, not perfection. And progress, my friends, is what sustains health."

—Donna Hanes, MD, University of Maryland Medical Center

"*Get a Move On!* is just what I need to help me get active once again. It's a mindset that helps me become more active in my everyday life. Thank you, Luisa Heymann!"

—Angeline Beach, retired Lockheed Martin executive

"If you want to shape up but don't even know where or how to start, this great little book will help you get moving. Incidentally, this is the only 'fitness' book that ever made me laugh out loud."

—David Kerns, author of *Fortnight on Maxwell Street* and *Standard of Care*

"What I love about this book is that it speaks to real people like the busy executives and entrepreneurial women that I coach who lament not having enough time in the day to engage in self-care. As a practitioner of somatic coaching, I stress the importance of exercise for anyone who wants to be successful! I will be adding this book to the toolkit that I offer clients."

—Nicole Cutts, PhD, success coach and clinical psychologist

"If, like me, you yearn to get fit but can't find the time to make it happen, then Luisa Heymann's new book, *Get a Move On!* was written just for you. Who knew that a little bit of effort invested in Mini-Workouts throughout the day could produce maximum results? Heymann's advice is simple, sensible, and—most of all—it's DO-able. She guides the reader through an instructive explanation of how she developed her methods and gives very specific examples of how to piggyback Mini-Workouts with almost any activity or environment in a normal day: cooking, sleeping, sex, driving, shopping, and even couch-potatoing! An inspiring book for anyone who wants to get fit without getting physical at the gym. Highly recommended."

—Morrie Warshawski, arts consultant and author, *Shaking the Money Tree*, *The Fundraising Houseparty*, and *this afternoon: 30 poems*

"*Get a Move On!* is a fantastic read. It is so much more than a motivational exercise book or program. It's a healthy perspective of incorporating exercise into your life anywhere at any time. No pressure, just do something. As a self-mastery mindset coach myself, I love this perspective, because for the first time this author doesn't make exercise a chore requiring a huge block of time in your schedule. This is a must-read... especially for all those women who think they just don't have time."

—Robin Joy Meyers, molecular geneticist, joy architect, TEDx and international speaker, author and self-mastery mindset coach

GET A MOVE ON!

Mini-Workouts Anytime, Anywhere

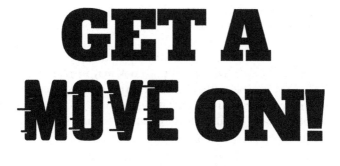

Luisa Coll-Pardo Heymann

Bold Story Press
Washington, DC

Bold Story Press, Washington, DC 20016
www.boldstorypress.com

First edition published July 2021

Printed in the United States of America
10 9 8 7 6 5 4 3 2 1

ISBN: 978-1-954805-00-2 (paperback)
ISBN: 978-1-954805-01-9 (e-book)

Library of Congress Control Number: 2021909403

Back cover: Photo by Sally Seymour, Seymour & Macintosh Photog-
raphy, Napa, California, https://www.seymourandmcintosh.com/

This book is dedicated...

to the drunk who passed out at the wheel in 2014 and totaled my car...if I'd never had a broken neck, I never would have written this book...

to John who has loved me because he thinks I'm interesting and beautiful whether I'm fit or flabby, thin or chubby, wearing sweatpants or a velvet gown...

to all the adults who corrected my English constantly, but still laughed at my made-up words...

to my sister Anne who came after me with a fly-swatter when she was two and I was new (though we eventually became pals)...

to the friends and family who—each in their own way— have supported, annoyed, and/or challenged me until I found my inner steel and outer calm...

and to all the folks who want to be healthier but who don't know where to begin...this book is for you; I hope it doesn't take a car wreck for you to find the motivation to find your fit.

Contents

CHAPTER 5
The Movements 57

CHAPTER 6
Mini-Workouts: Adding It All Up 73

CHAPTER 7
What Exercising Does for Your Body

Introduction

I'm hardly an Olympic-level athlete (I spend a lot of time at my desk and love to binge-watch mysteries), but I like to hike and am such a water-baby that I taught aqua aerobics for 20+ years, so I've always managed to stay in reasonably good shape...sometimes better, sometimes worse, but consistently pretty energetic and healthy, even if my weight has been like a yo-yo ever since high school.

Then in 2014, I was sidelined with a broken neck after being hit by a drunk driver—ouch!—and in a nanosecond, my life was turned upside down.

For months I was in a neck brace and could barely move, so when I was finally able to resume something approaching normal life, I had to start getting back into shape in teeny-tiny bite-sized pieces; thus, the concept of Mini-Workouts was born. By consistently doing Mini-Workouts every day, gradually increasing repetitions and upping the number of daily sessions as I was able, I eventually found my way back to good health. I was lucky...and I was very persistent. I soon realized that Mini-Workouts were a fantastic addition to my weekly schedule, even once I could exercise normally again, and have kept it up ever since. Some days I'm really disciplined and highly motivated; other days I phone it in (hey, I'm no angel), but I do at least some, every single day, and it pays huge dividends in terms of strength and stamina and good health, considering the minimal effort required.

If you're in a similar situation working to come back from an illness or injury, are sedentary and would like to have more energy, have a scary health problem that you need to get under control, or are just plain tired of being out of shape and don't know where or how to begin to get your body on the road to better health, Mini-Workouts are a great place to start.

How much time do you spend each day idly waiting for something to happen? I'll show you how you can use that time to start getting some tone in your muscles and maybe even some control over your life.

Let's see what you could do with the 30-60-90 or more seconds you currently spend staring at the microwave waiting for it to beep, or what you might do (that's more productive than swearing) when stuck in traffic.

P.S. Mini-Workouts are kind of fun, too.

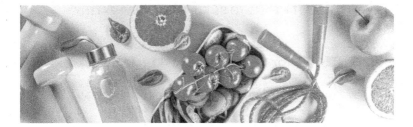

CHAPTER 1

What It Means to Be Fit, Well, and Healthy

Here in the US, we typically talk about fitness in terms of athletic ability, but having a healthy body has very little to do with dunking baskets, running races, or whacking balls. Overall fitness and wellness are composed of several different components, all of which play a vital role in your health picture, and these are determined by how much you move and the food choices you make day in/day out, week in/week out, year in/year out—not by occasional weekend warrior activities or once-in-a-blue-moon binges.

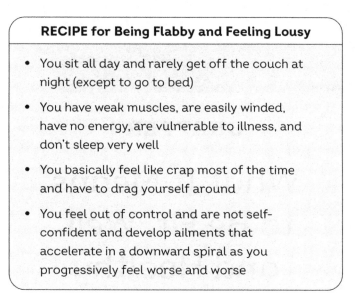

RECIPE for Being Flabby and Feeling Lousy

- You sit all day and rarely get off the couch at night (except to go to bed)

- You have weak muscles, are easily winded, have no energy, are vulnerable to illness, and don't sleep very well

- You basically feel like crap most of the time and have to drag yourself around

- You feel out of control and are not self-confident and develop ailments that accelerate in a downward spiral as you progressively feel worse and worse

Of course, it also helps *a lot* if you eat a wide variety of nutritious foods so your body has the fuel it needs to function properly—not to mention you'd be doing yourself a tremendous favor if you stopped consuming the many popular sugar-fat-salt-chemical food and drink bombs that throw your whole system out of whack and pack on unwanted pounds—but let's tackle one thing at a time, namely figuring out how *you* can organize *your* schedule and establish helpful habits to benefit *your* health, now and in the future.

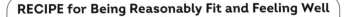

RECIPE for Being Reasonably Fit and Feeling Well

- You move enough that your body can easily perform normal activities

- You have fewer aches and pains and sleep better, so you're more alert and your body is better able to fend off illness

- Because you are healthier, you have a more positive outlook and have sufficient energy for work and play, so you enjoy life more

- You have the stamina to accomplish what you need to get done each day

- You feel more self-confident and in control of your life as you reinforce the habits that keep you feeling well because it's oh-so-much-better than the negative cycle described above

THE PURSUIT OF WELLNESS

Being really well inside and outside—that is to say happy and healthy—is multilayered, individual, and complicated, but the simple fact of the matter is that when you're upbeat and energetic, you attract optimistic people and affirmative outcomes to yourself in ways that are self-reinforcing. But you've got to prime the pump, so to speak, by doing what it takes to get yourself into a positive state of well-being in the first place, or at least clearly headed in that direction. The elements of wellness are frequently described as an absence of disease, an absence of chronic pain, regularly getting sufficient rejuvenating sleep, feeling energetic, having a positive mental outlook, and having some sense of control over your life. It's interesting to note that much of what comprises the concept of wellness is simply an absence of ailments, and it is instructive to remember that many common ailments are directly caused by a lack of adequate nutrition and the habitual consumption of foods that actually make you ill, frequently coupled with a sedentary lifestyle.

Most fitness books urge you to immediately sign up for hours of weekly aerobics classes and/or adopt an exercise schedule that may be completely unrealistic given your current obligations, schedule, ability, and/or health picture. In the past, I have often bought magazines with articles about people who've lost tons of weight—you've undoubtedly seen them lined up at the checkout stands and probably bought them, too—the covers invariably have pictures of thin people standing inside their old jeans with screaming headlines like:

"Half Their Size!!!"

But when I read about how many hours a day these people spend taking exercise classes and what they typically eat, I think, *forget it*, because I know I'm not going to dedicate every waking hour to being at the gym and, frankly, I'd rather die young than eat nothing but steamed vegetables for the rest of my life. So, what to do?

If you try to follow a program that requires too many changes in too short a period of time, it's inevitable you'll abandon it. Instead of throwing yourself into a repeat of the *Get Magically Fit in X-Number of Weeks for a New Improved You!* that wasn't successful or sustainable the last time you tried it, let's try a completely different approach that will allow you to make progress quickly enough that you won't get discouraged, but doesn't require you to completely change your life and lifestyle overnight.

Get a Move On! is a practical guide to help you reasonably incorporate small changes into your daily routines that can make a very big difference in your well-being without totally disrupting your current schedule. You can be measurably healthier, fitter, and thinner—plus have a more positive outlook on life—by regularly moving enough to improve muscle tone and give your body and brain the oxygen needed to function at a halfway decent level. That's right…

Our intention here is to be in moderately decent shape and noticeably less flabby and jiggly.

For those of you who are sedentary couch potatoes or semi-couch potatoes, Mini-Workouts can quickly put you on a path to feeling better and being healthier. In addition to being an ideal starting point for anyone whose normal activity level is the bare minimum, Mini-Workouts are also really useful for:

- People who already exercise a little who'd like to be a bit stronger and fitter, but won't or can't devote any more time to working out

- Those who exercise semi-regularly and would like to do better, but have a full schedule and simply don't have time for more

- Enthusiastic regular exercisers who'd like to be stronger, but are already stressing their joints to the max

If you fall into one of these three categories, you're already at least somewhat knowledgeable about exercising, so you'll easily be able to figure out which body part needs the most work and can tailor Mini-Workouts to focus on strengthening or stretching one or two targeted areas.

SITTING, INTERRUPTED

Students have to sit for much of the day; many jobs require being at a desk for hours at a stretch; and commutes typically entail being stuck in a small seat for a block of time as you get from home to school or work and back. Once home, you might need to spend time at your desk doing homework or sorting mail, or you may relax with your feet up while you read the news, catch up on social media, or maybe do some online shopping. Out of habit, you might just plop down in your favorite chair to unwind with a drink at the end of the day, whether it was a stressful day or not. All this (in)activity is usually followed by a short move to the kitchen or dining room where you are seated for dinner and then, worn out from a long day of mostly sitting, you collapse on the sofa to read or watch television... because all that sitting really and truly is exhausting!

The human body is not designed to sit still for hours and hours without moving, so even if you can't change your work or commute, if you want to feel well and be healthy, you must resolve to interrupt your chair-time and sofa-lounging at regular intervals; with a little organization and a bit of inspiration, you can easily accomplish this. Present-day technologies simultaneously allow and force us to save energy in almost all facets of our lives and though the benefits are many—I personally have no desire to hand-grind my own corn, nor does hauling water from the well hold any appeal—there's a physical cost to pay for modern conveniences as we become increasingly sedentary. For a fee, someone else will collect and deliver groceries to your doorstep, or even take your dog out for a poopertunity. Spurred on by COVID-19, internet shopping increased exponentially in 2020 and, though all pandemics eventually subside, online shopping is here to stay. Robots are moving in, time- and energy-saving appliances are commonplace, and drone deliveries will soon be ho-hum. Even little things like listening to music or switching lights on and off can now be accomplished by doing nothing more than speaking Alexa's name. With enough remote controls and voice-activated gizmos, we'll soon be able to run our entire households and accomplish all our chores while barely moving a muscle.

Until about a hundred years ago, people had to walk, run, bike, or ride a horse to get from one place to another, but now we mostly just sit in whatever conveyance is most convenient, and as self-driving cars become a reality, soon we won't even have to make the minimal effort required to drive. Common tasks such as typing have gotten so easy you barely have to do more than flutter your fingers, whereas a few generations ago at least you had to hit the carriage return lever and turn the platen, and it probably won't be long before artificial intelligence enables us to just speak to our computers and QWERTY will be as quaintly old-fashioned as a rotary-dial phone. In the past, you had to move at least some to manage the various aspects of everyday living, and even though many tasks hardly required what you'd call a big effort (like crossing the room to change the TV channel or walking down the hall to answer the phone), these thousands of little movements kept your muscles fired up all day. This is no longer true and if we're not careful, we can easily get to the point where we *can't* do things, because we *don't* do them on a regular basis.

Once, when I was a Peace Corps Volunteer in rural Costa Rica, I was helping host a group of visitors from the US who were touring our local agricultural high school. The program started around 9:00 a.m. and then we took a break at 10:30. Our guests assumed we were taking a coffee and donuts kind of break and were rather shocked to realize we were breaking for lunch and that lunch consisted of a giant plate of rice and beans with an egg and vegetables and chicken and salad, followed by cake. One of the visitors whispered her surprise that everyone was chowing down like that at such an early hour and asked if this was normal. I replied that, yes, all but the cake was typical; the cake was in their honor as a special treat. Before I could say more, she wondered aloud how they could all be so trim and fit if they ate like that all the time...because it wasn't in her frame of reference to think that everyone else had already put in two or three hours of physical labor before the program started and would put in three more before taking an afternoon siesta and then four or five more before heading home for dinner, and that on the weekend, they'd play soccer for fun and if there was a wedding, they'd play music and dance until the wee hours.

There's an excellent book by Daniel Lieberman, *Exercised: Why Something We Never Evolved to Do Is Healthy and Rewarding*, that explains how and why humans aren't inclined to spend calories needlessly, aka exercising, because just doing what's required to survive in a non-modern society takes all the calorie input that most people can get. Given the option, the *campesinos* in my Costa Rican town would lie in bed or slouch in a chair, too—a torrential downpour was often viewed with immense pleasure—but in their world, a day of inactivity is a rarity. In other words, if you dislike exerting yourself unless there's a concrete reward attached, you're not alone. If there's a choice between expending energy and taking advantage of an opportunity to rest, it is easy—and so tempting—and utterly rational—and completely normal—to want to veg out in a comfy chair. Back in the good old/bad old days, if you wanted to eat you had to work—whatever you wanted to accomplish, from the largest to the smallest activity, required you to move.

As our opportunities to be sedentary have increased, as a nation we have become flabbier, weaker, and generally less healthy, and inadequate movement coupled with the constant availability of low-nutrition/high-calorie foods, has brought us to the point where there is an epidemic of obesity with the attendant ailments of diabetes, high blood pressure, heart disease, gout, breathing problems, etc. Most of us are fully aware which of our body parts need work, and the desire to be healthier, stronger, more energetic, and to feel more attractive drives a continuing search for self-improvement (and/or constant self-recrimination, even though that's not especially helpful unless it spurs us to action). It's not surprising that there's a steady supply of new programs, ideas, gadgets, and pills to help us achieve these goals, and many offer the promise of miraculous quick-fixes because, yes, it would certainly be nice to achieve instant good health and fitness without making any effort.

When embarking on your new "I've really, really, really gotta get in shape" program, start with a modest goal for minor improvement. You can't make up for years of inactivity with a few intense sessions of crazy, go-for-broke, exhausting exercise, as that will surely lead to pain or injury and leave you feeling frustrated. Instead, aim for a reachable target of making a few small changes every week that will steadily produce slow but noticeable, measurable, sustainable benefits (specific tips on how you can do this are what follows in the rest of this book). Recognize that the human body is not designed for sitting undisturbed for numerous hours in a row and that if you force yours to do something so unnatural, it will cease to function properly.

MAKE FRIENDS WITH YOUR BODY...FOR LIFE

Remind yourself every day that your body is not your enemy, but the cherished house in which your spirit resides. Make a conscious effort to nurture a sense of gratitude for the way it responds to requests (pick up the fork/kick the ball/roll over) and all the things it does without you even having to ask (pump blood/expand and contract the lungs/ grow fingernails). Do you hate your house just because it has a stair that creaks? Of course not, you just recognize that as one of its quirks. If your roof leaks, you don't despise the house for the leak—you do what you can to fix it, right? Can you show the same acceptance and consideration toward your body that you show toward your house?

Despite relentless cultural pressure to spend your money to meet someone else's ideal of beauty, give yourself permission to love and cherish yourself. If you think your thighs are too flabby, instead of hating them, just ask yourself what you can do to make them stronger (walk more, do leg lifts) and thank them for being able to take you from Point A to Point B which is, after all, their primary purpose.

Do you have a body part that's broken, like maybe an arm that doesn't function right? Strengthen it if you can. Thank it for what it can do. Forgive it for what it can't. Treat yourself with at least as much kindness and sympathy as you would show to a complete stranger.

Does the idea of self-love seem too touchy-feely for you to even contemplate or have you hated some body part for so long you can't quite shift your thinking? Start by finding one or two things to love about your body and then next week, find another. Start a sentence with the words "I love..." and then finish it with something affirming. Several years ago, I was at a conference where we did this exercise and here's the list I started with: I love having the red hair that runs in our family, because it connects us to each other and our Scottish ancestors. I love my hands, despite the wrinkles, because I have great manual dexterity. I love having the same gray-blue-green eyes that my grandfather had. I love the high arches of my beautiful feet that look great in sandals!

Start your own list today and if you usually say something like, "I hate my thighs," instead say something like, "I love my: strong hands / freckled nose / infectious laugh / curly hair / excellent eye-sight / keen sense of smell / long neck / and beautiful smile."

Show yourself some compassion. Forgive your body for its imperfections (perceived or real) and hold it in the high esteem that it deserves…it's the only one you'll ever have.

Forget the pie-in-the-sky images that are so often dangled before your eyes—usually with the "promise" that if you'd only do one secret thing or send someone a wad of your hard-earned money, you'll miraculously lose weight and look like Venus or Adonis—and recognize that you won't be a Lycra-clad model with six-pack abs or be showing off a tight size two bum in stretchy white jeans any time soon unless you're currently a size four. If you're hoping for dramatic weight loss like you might see on a TV show like *The Biggest Loser*, keep in mind that many of the contestants on the show took diet pills that made them ill, vomited on a regular basis, and—despite all this— regained most of the weight lost during the show in the months that followed, mainly because they hadn't developed healthy and sustainable eating and exercising habits, and/or ate so few calories that they completely screwed up their metabolisms so that their body went into starvation mode protecting its stored fat. You won't achieve a perfect "pre-baby weight" body three months after giving birth unless, like the celebrities featured in magazine articles, you have a private trainer and personal chef at your beck and call. I suggest you ignore or throw away anything that uses the word "skinny" to define your ultimate goal... healthy people are not skinny, they are medium-sized (I almost called this book *The Happy Medium* until I realized it sounded like a book about a jolly psychic). Envision yourself just a little bit stronger and a little bit healthier and a little bit slimmer. Hold a picture in your mind of a slightly healthier version of who you are right now, and let that picture be target number one. Remember, comparing yourself to a supermodel or professional athlete is just setting yourself up for failure and disappointment.

> *Your goal is to be the best possible*
> *you...everyone else is already taken.*
> —Oscar Wilde
>
> Irish poet, playwright,
> novelist, and
> internationally famous wit

CHAPTER 2

Realistic Assessment and Goal-Setting

Without putting any value judgment on where you are now, make an honest assessment of your current level of fitness, wellness, and/or health challenges, and then identify what would be for you—that's you, not anyone else—a modest improvement, and set that as your first goal.

Chances are good you have a vague desire to "lose weight" and "be healthier," but instead of picking an arbitrary number on the scale as something to shoot for (as you've probably done many times before), identify something specific that will improve your health and quality of life, such as:

- Being able to go up a flight of stairs without becoming winded

- Having sufficient arm strength to pick up suitcases or groceries without struggling

- Bringing your cholesterol level down out of the danger zone

- Feeling like you can say "yes" when invited to participate in an activity you like

- Lowering blood pressure enough to substantially reduce the risk of a heart attack

- Having enough energy to ride a bicycle or skateboard

- Preventing pre-diabetes from becoming full-blown diabetes (80% of all adults with diabetes are medically overweight or obese and get very little exercise)

- Being able to go on a favorite hike with friends

- Getting (back) into shape so you can go dancing or play tennis

- Reducing stiffness or pain from arthritis
- Being fit enough to enjoy a camping trip
- Feeling well enough to play with your children or grandchildren or the family dog

Once you've identified the general nature of your goal, start to flesh out the details and/or set a timeline so you know what success will look like. For example, if your current cholesterol count is dangerously high, it would be great if you could reduce it by 10 or 15 percent in a month or two. Hurrah! Big improvement! When you've got that success under your belt, you can set a new target number as the next goal, but if you'll only feel successful if you can reduce it by 25 percent in two or three weeks, you'll give up because that's an unrealistic goal that's not even remotely attainable.

If your goal is being able to go up a flight of stairs without becoming winded, get specific about which stairs you're talking about—the stairs at your office or school? The ones at your house or apartment? Climbing the steps of a ladder to clean the gutters? The stairs at the mall? The Spanish Steps in Rome? The stairs at your local sports arena to get up to the sky-high bleacher seats?

Here's an example of how a "stair goal" can work: There's a great seafood restaurant in Seattle's Pike Place called Lowell's, where the kitchen is downstairs and the dining room is up; consequently, as you might imagine, the entire waitstaff has rock-hard thighs and buns, but they certainly didn't all start out that way. On one visit, our server, who was working during his summer break from school, told us that in order to prepare for the job, he'd started taking the stairs wherever he could for months in advance. Initially, he was huffing and puffing and would have to stop once or twice to rest when he took the stairs at his apartment building. More than once he thought about looking for a more sedentary job, but he had friends who worked at Lowell's and the money was good, so he kept at it and just kept using the stairs everywhere he went. By the time the job started, he could manage the numerous trips without too much trouble: up/down, up/down, up/down, although his coworkers would fly past him. After a couple of months, he was zooming up and down with the best of them, and he really enjoyed it. He told us he'd already signed on to work there the following summer so he'll have motivation to keep taking the stairs all year, because he's in the best shape of his life and he's really happy about it.

If a lengthy bike ride is your long-term goal, start with a short-term objective of riding one or two miles or even one or two blocks or maybe just five minutes on a stationary bike. Do whatever you can successfully accomplish that moves you in the right direction, even if it's not a lot, and then celebrate when you reach your limited but doable goal. Every time you hit a target, you can set another one and keep doing that until you arrive at your ultimate goal…but take time to give yourself a big pat on the back for reaching the first one and give yourself permission to feel good about it, even if you're still far short of your ideal.

A good example of the successful achievement of a series of reachable goals is my not-so-young friend Scott, who has always loved cycling, but couldn't ride at all after knee surgery. Additionally, he'd been unable to exercise much in general for quite a while beforehand due to knee pain, so he had steadily become weaker and flabbier. When he finally healed enough post-surgery to do more than just the most basic physical therapy, he rode a stationary bike one minute, twice a day. Yep, one minute, a measly 60 seconds. As he felt progressively better, he upped the sessions to two minutes; soon it was five minutes three times a day. A few weeks later it was 10, a couple more it was 15…and he celebrated his success at each stage, not just when he was finally able to ride long distances with his buddies again. He didn't sit on the couch all day bemoaning the fact that he wasn't strong enough to go on his favorite rides, but did what he could to make slow, steady, gradual, measurable progress toward his longer-term goal. A year and a half later, Scott won first place in his age-category for a long-distance bike race, but he was proud of his accomplishments every day, every step of the way, not just when he finally crossed the finish line. Those initial 60-second rides had taken more guts and determination than any of the fun rides he took when he felt well.

Right about now you may be thinking, I have zero interest in any kind of race, biking or otherwise, so what does this have to do with me? For every person like Scott, there are many thousands more who will never set a goal of winning any kind of athletic competition. Nevertheless, whether you define it this way or not, and whether you like it or not, you are in a race against creeping decrepitude every single day of your life and the long-term goal is to be a healthy adult who can enjoy life well into old age.

It's a constant competition with yourself: Should I watch TV or go for a walk? Read more news or do yoga? Look at celebrity pix or ride my bike? Flip through a magazine or take an exercise class? Life is often a lot like the cartoons that show a little devil on one shoulder and an angel on the other...whispering in your ears with opposing instructions: "C'mon! One more cat video, what can it hurt?" versus "Put on some sneakers and go for a walk! You know you'll feel better if you get up and move." If necessary, promise yourself a reward or find images to plant in your brain of a desired or feared outcome—whatever motivates you best. Some people respond better to a carrot than a stick, and you may have to think about what truly motivates you. If you don't want to spend time dissecting the factors that drive your behaviors, then just remind yourself every day...

MOVE IT AND USE IT–OR LOSE IT

One 80-something I know has a goal of staying out of a wheelchair, and that's her motivation to get up and move every day, even when she doesn't feel like it. She keeps very clear, very different scenarios in her head: one of herself continuing to volunteer at a museum she loves, seeing her friends at the pool where she takes a class, and going out for a meal or a movie when she feels like it, and the other of herself in a wheelchair, waiting for the handicap-access van, only being able to go places when it's convenient for someone else to accompany her. She knows all too well that this second possibility is the reality for many sedentary older adults.

When it comes to self-assessment and goal setting, I highly recommend that you follow this outstanding advice from writer Charles L. Bosk as you think about your future self, how you want to live, and who you want to become.

FORGIVE AND REMEMBER

That's right: forgive and remember, not forgive and forget. If you rarely move more than is absolutely necessary, have flabby weak muscles, and/or are hauling around a lot of extra weight, remember that this less-than-ideal state of health didn't just suddenly appear out of the blue, nor is it the result of one week of being particularly lazy...or two weeks of crazy bingeing...or a month of too much partying...but rather the gradual loss of muscle tone and/or the accumulation of excess fat caused by too much sitting around in combination with too many calories consumed on a regular basis over a very l-o-o-o-o-n-g period of time (probably years).

It may be that you're surrounded by people who never want to do anything but watch television, so you do too, or maybe you were raised by people who gave you lots of sugary treats and too few vegetables. You may have been persuaded by relentless advertising that in order to "be cool" you must drink soft drinks constantly and have now become addicted to them (why not? they have the best ad campaigns in the world and you are exposed to them constantly) so you have gained a lot of weight and feel jittery and/or sluggish much of the time. Perhaps you have a slow metabolism and are inclined to be sedentary or it could be that you have a body type that stores fat easily and releases it only begrudgingly (no, the genetic lottery is not fair). Maybe you were sidelined at some point with an illness or injury and gained a lot of weight and that started you on the path to becoming a couch potato. If you suffered trauma as a kid, you might have reacted by unconsciously but deliberately overeating until you ate yourself sick and stopped going outside to play; additionally, many school districts have cut out physical education, so you might be stuck in a chair all day, even if you'd rather be outside getting some exercise and doing something fun. It could be that you love your digital devices so much you've given up all other activities in order to sit on your duff and stare at a screen all day...if so, you've certainly got plenty of company in that regard.

Whatever your current situation may be, think about how you got to where you are now and be specific about the behaviors that have robbed you of good health.

Now forgive yourself for how you got here. Maybe the fact that you're unhealthy and/or flabby and/or overweight is your own damned fault and maybe it isn't, but however you arrived at your current state of not-so-great health, show some compassion and forgive yourself. If necessary, scream and yell! Stomp your feet! Throw a tantrum! And then forgive yourself (and others, if you can...you don't have to like them, but holding onto anger hurts you, not them) and make a conscious decision to move on and replace the unhealthy choices that have become your pattern with choices that will put you on the road to better health.

Picture yourself in three months, then six, in one year or five or 10, at age 40 or 60 or 90, and ask: How do I want to feel then? What do I want to be able to do? Where do I want to go? Am I making choices every day that move me toward my goals?

Whatever happened in the past—good, bad, or indifferent—is now irrevocably done with, finished, over and unchangeable, and regardless of how you got to where you are now, it's an absolute certainty that...

Until you stop wishing for a different past,
it will be impossible to craft a healthy future.

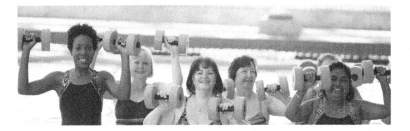

CHAPTER 3

The Elements of Fitness and Mini-Workouts

Fitness is about being sufficiently coordinated and strong enough to meet the physical challenges of moving through the world and being able to easily accomplish what you need and want to do—in other words, enough pep for both work and play. Rather than aiming for some ideal of buff, athletic perfection that will inevitably lead to disappointment, let's look at how you can be in moderately good shape by tweaking and adjusting your lifestyle, without totally disrupting it, by putting what is currently just wasted time to good use.

Discussions around "getting fitter" usually revolve around setting up an exercise class schedule and adding sports and other activities to your weekly routine. These are valuable (and fun), and we'll look at some practical ways you might do this further along, but the focus here is on incorporating movement routines into your everyday schedule in bite-sized sessions that can add up to make an incredible difference. You can start right now—no equipment needed, no money required, you don't even have to wear shoes. I call them:

MINI-WORKOUTS

Mini-Workouts are quick sets of exercises that you link to activities that are already part of your everyday life. For the most part, they don't add any time to your schedule, but are something useful you can do while you are waiting…waiting…waiting…waiting…waiting… for something or someone. In a few cases, you might add a few seconds or a minute here or there to a regularly performed activity, but in no case do these take up a big chunk of time.

Being as strong as an Olympian may not be in your near future, but kind of fit and way less jiggly are absolutely within reach. You can start to see noticeable improvements in muscle tone very quickly with very modest but consistent—repeat, consistent—effort. If you incorporate Mini-Workouts into your regular routine and commit yourself to doing them absolutely every day, you will see real progress within weeks. Additionally, if you've been totally or somewhat sedentary for a long time and start a walking program, even a very limited one, you will likely soon feel better than you have in a long time, your health numbers will improve, and excess weight will slowly but surely start to melt away (more on practical ways to fit that into your schedule later).

THE SIX ELEMENTS OF FITNESS

Rather than assessing fitness in the usual way by asking how strong, fast, muscular, and thin you are, let's look at it a little differently by examining six basic physical attributes:

1. **Aerobic Fitness (cardio)** = healthy lungs and heart = stamina

2. **Core Strength** = stability and good body alignment + a stronger back, less prone to aches and pains

3. **Muscle Mass and Strength** = ability to lift, push, and pull + burn more calories even at rest

4. **Flexibility** = full range of motion + suppleness and fluidity of movement

5. **Coordination** = accuracy of motion and reaction speed

6. **Balance** = being sure on your feet and avoiding falls

Most of us are stronger in one area than another and you should tailor your routines to improve where you are weak and work to maintain or improve where you're already doing reasonably well. A quick look around any mall, stadium, gym, or airport will show you a variety of different body types and combinations, many of which are headed for potentially serious health problems: the graceful woman who danced as a girl but is now carrying an extra 60 or 80 pounds (maybe has adult-onset diabetes, and could lose a toe or foot one day); the overweight teenagers drinking sodas and eating pizza while watching videos of other people playing sports (may be truly obese by their 20s and in danger of a heart attack by age 40); the super muscular guy who lifts weights all the time, but is clumsy and lacks balance (could be at a high risk of a fall at some point); the nervous person who is thin but flabby and lives on sweets (has low bone density and bad teeth, may be headed for kidney failure and possibly a future hip fracture); the pregnant-looking man who played football in high school and still eats like he's burning 7,000 calories a day on the field (has high blood pressure and may be headed for a stroke)…and on and on. How would you describe yourself if you could see yourself from afar?

Do an honest self-assessment, then celebrate where you're strong and give yourself a kick in the pants to get moving on the areas where there's room for improvement.

MINI-WORKOUTS
CHANGE YOUR BODY AND BRAIN

The key to success is to connect a specific Mini-Workout to a specific regular daily activity and then every time you perform that activity, it triggers you to do your quick exercise routine. You may have to force yourself to do Mini-Workouts every day for a week, and then remind yourself to do them every week for a month, and then before you know it, you'll just do them every day without thinking about it, because it's your habit to do so. As former Olympic track and field champion Jim Ryun said, "Motivation is what gets you started; habit is what keeps you going." The habit of Mini-Workouts can pay significant health dividends in a number of different ways:

- Mini-Workouts help keep you brighter and more energetic during the course of the day because each one sends oxygen to your brain and "wakes up" your little gray cells.

- After you've successfully done three or five or twenty Mini-Workouts in a day, you'll probably want to walk more, or may even get motivated to swing by the gym.

- You avoid the common problem of extended periods of complete inactivity—notably sitting for hours and hours—which in addition to causing stiffness, soreness, and weight gain, has been shown to be extremely exceptionally extraordinarily bad for health (some say too much sitting is as detrimental to health as smoking).

- Throughout the day, they serve as reminders that you care about your health, so you may be more likely to reach for a piece of fruit instead of a piece of cake.

- If you miss a scheduled walk or skip an exercise class for some reason, at least you never get to the end of a day having done absolutely nothing, zero, zip, zilch, nada.

- After each Mini-Workout you get to feel a bit virtuous, a lovely feeling that makes you feel good about yourself and have a more positive outlook.

In the following chapters, there are lists of some common daily activities with suggestions for creating Mini-Workout routines to link to them and detailed descriptions of various exercise options. If a physical limitation prevents you from doing a suggested exercise, then do something else—but do something.

For exercise newbies, a "routine" is a series of exercises done one after another and a "set" is the number of repetitions ("reps" in gym lingo) of a particular exercise done at one go. If you do three sets of 10 reps, it means there's a rest between sets, and the total number of repetitions is 30.

Some of the movements are suggested as freestanding exercises, but if necessary, rest a hand on a counter, wall, or the back of a sturdy chair for support (not a rolling chair, please don't be a nominee for the Darwin Awards). Start with a number of repetitions that you can do comfortably and then gradually increase that number, pushing yourself to do a couple more and then a few more, little by little.

It's truly amazing how much exercise Mini-Workouts can provide over the course of a week and you will notice small but definite improvements very quickly. In Chapter 6, there are cumulative calculations that will probably astound you.

> *If you don't like the road you're walking, start paving another one.*
>
> —Dolly Parton
>
> Singer, songwriter, musician, record producer, actress, author, businesswoman, and philanthropist

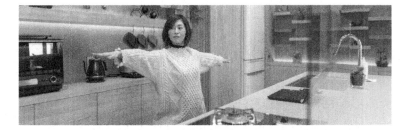

CHAPTER 4

Link Your Daily Activities to Mini-Workouts

Please note that kitchens and bathrooms can be dangerous places—you may have room for marching in place, modified wall push-ups, or bicep curls but not leg lifts or swimming moves—so use common sense and adapt your routines to fit the space.

TURNING EVERYDAY TASKS INTO "ME" TIME

We humans are hardwired to conserve our physical energy so we have reserves to run like hell in case a saber-toothed tiger decides we look like dinner. Once you recognize that we are all predisposed by nature to be sedentary when we get the chance—and that this impulse is no longer especially valid for most of us in our modern world where our well-being is more likely to be threatened by a box of donuts than T. Rex—you can start to identify the numerous opportunities you have every day to either stay still as you wait for something to happen, or view these blocks of time as a chance to move in ways that will provide small but regular health benefits.

Humans also protect their energy reserves by establishing regular patterns of behavior in order to keep from becoming exhausted by decision-making about repetitive occurrences. Imagine how worn out you'd be before you even left home if each day you had to decide anew if you should wash your face or brush your teeth first, or whether you should put the milk in your cup before or after the coffee...or if you'd maybe prefer tea and, if so, do you want lemon, etc. Since we all have limited bandwidth, we must reserve our brainpower to deal with whatever is new, unexpected, or threatening. In the 21st century, we don't need to worry too much about a new species of pterodactyl showing up, but the speed at which things change in the internet age means we need to pace ourselves and establish routines in order to be able to process a constant barrage of new information. Once a habit is well established—whether good, bad, or indifferent— keeping up with it becomes as second nature and easy as putting on socks before shoes, but frequent repetitions are required to get to that point. There are descriptions below of commonplace activities and ideas for routines you can link to them, but feel free to make up your own to fit into the flow of your day, as long as whatever you choose can be repeated on a daily basis. If you regularly perform your Mini-Workout routines at the same time and/or in the same place, they will soon become ingrained habit.

In the Kitchen

Waiting…waiting…waiting: Waiting for a pan to heat or food to cook, for a pot to boil, the microwave to beep, the ice to dispense, the blender to whirl, the water pitcher to fill, the tap to get hot, waiting for toast, toasting nuts, stirring, grinding, processing, perking, puréeing, and many etceteras. We probably spend more time in the kitchen waiting for something to happen than anywhere else, so why waste all that time? The waiting is usually done in short bursts, but these add up over the course of a week, even if you're not much of a cook. While you're waiting, do any freestanding movements (e.g., marching in place, toe-touches) or those where you need a counter for balance (leg lifts); any appropriate arm exercises (overhead reaches, swimming strokes, isometric hand presses); stretching moves (calf stretch, hand flexes, shoulder rolls); or try some dance moves like the Twist, the Macarena, or...maybe a little Funky Chicken while waiting for your oatmeal? You get the idea.

In the Bathroom

- Standing at the sink brushing your teeth: Any standing leg exercises (lean against the counter or hold on with one hand for balance if needed). Too uncoordinated? Maybe just march in place or rise up on your toes.

- While drying your hair, using a towel, or rubbing in lotion: Side-step-slide and march in place.

- Waiting for the water to get hot in the shower: If your shower has a step threshold (and you have tile that's not slippery and something to hold onto), step up and down or do any other step aerobics moves you know; if no step, do any standing leg exercises or arm movements.

- Waiting for the tub to fill: Use the five or ten minutes to do any routines you have room for—why just stand there staring at the tap? If it's really slow, throw a towel or mat on a nearby floor and do butt-squeezes or floor exercises (just don't let the tub overflow).

- Sitting on the toilet: Any seated exercises, appropriate arm exercises, or easy stretches.

- After you've used the toilet: Close the lid, then do a set of squat/sit/stands every time you go and keep increasing your repetitions. If a urinal is your only option or using a toilet with the lid closed won't work for whatever reason, go find a nearby chair or bench, but make the link between going to the bathroom and squat/sit/stands inextricable because everyone uses the bathroom numerous times every day.

- After you wash your hands: Do some overhead arm reaches or torso twists, and maybe a few shoulder rolls.

In the Bedroom

- Just after waking, before getting out of bed: Loosen up your body by wiggling toes and fingers and take a few deep breaths. With straight legs, tighten thigh muscles and hold for a few seconds (do a Kegel* contraction at the same time); repeat 5–10 times. Flex feet up and down 5–10 times, followed by ankle rolls in, then out, followed by 10 or more butt squeezes. With legs straight, slide one foot up to a bent knee position then straighten, 10–20 repetitions; do the other leg; do both legs together. With feet together and knees bent, do a few bridge lifts while contracting your abs. If you're inclined, lift both legs straight up in the air with heels together, separate heels until making a wide vee, then heels back together; follow this by hugging knees to chest. Big yawn (enough to stretch your face muscles); get up and start the day with purpose.

- Getting dressed: This is a great time to work on balance. While perusing your closet or dresser trying to decide what to wear, stand on one leg, lift your arms up in the air and hold for a moment. When you lift your foot to step into pants, slow the process w-a-a-ay down so you balance on one foot for a moment or two (hold on or lean against something if needed). Lift one knee and point and flex your foot with arms out for balance or use the time to just march in place or step side-to-side.

- Doing routine chores like making the bed or changing the sheets: Put on some salsa music, dance around, and make a game out of it (e.g., lift pillows front/overhead/side-to-side before putting them in place or do overhead arm reaches or toe touches after tucking in the sheet).

- Having sex: If your sex life is great, get more athletic, try new positions, make it last longer. If your sex life is boring and you normally just lie there and "think of England" as the Victorians used to recommend, work on stomach crunches, hip lifts, and stretch a bit—at least it won't be a complete waste of time and, who knows, maybe you'll even start to have more fun.

In the Office or at Your Desk

- On the phone: When possible, get up and walk around the room (use the speaker or invest in a wireless earpiece). If walking around isn't possible, just stand up and shift from one foot to the other. When stuck in the chair, tap your feet, alternate lifting your heels and toes, do leg raises, and switch the phone from one ear to the other occasionally to do some arm exercises. If you're on a conference call where you're just listening, put the phone on mute (in case you grunt, how rude) and do your squat/sit/stand routine and arm exercises, swivel around in your chair, and do seated leg exercises (make sure your chair is stable and doesn't roll out from under you).

- Using the computer: Think of what you can do while your computer boots up (lots, depending on connection speed). While working, rather than leaving your hand poised on the mouse or track pad, it's better to click and then take your hand away immediately and make it a habit, as not only does this leave your hands and arms free to do some exercises, it helps prevent stiffness and/or carpal tunnel syndrome. You can do any of the exercises mentioned in the "Sitting on the Toilet" section, plus use your legs to roll your chair back and forth or swivel side-to-side and do the seated abdominal workout. You can still read or type while you're doing these—I know, I'm doing little crunches right now.

- Extended time at the desk: In addition to the moves mentioned above, get up at least every 20 or 30 minutes and go do something. Get a glass of water or cup of coffee, make some copies, go talk to someone in person instead of sending a text or IM. Use a bathroom that's not close by, and if you're in a multi-floor building, get in the habit of using facilities on a different floor and take the stairs. If you can, go outside from time to time to stretch your legs and get some fresh air, as even a brief respite is better than none at all.

In the Car or on the Bus, Subway, or Train

While obviously limited by space constraints, you can still move around at least some. If you're the driver, you can do butt squeezes any time and when stopped in traffic you can use the time to do seated leg exercises, isometric arm exercises, and any other simple arm exercises you have room for (and maybe will feel less stressed-out about getting stuck at a light). If you're a passenger, you can do these plus seated abdominal crunches.

Taking a Lunch Break

When possible, walk to restaurants and to run errands. If you've brought your lunch, walk around before and after eating (up and down stairs, up and down the hall, around the block, to your car, just think of something that gets you moving and make it your new routine).

If you have regular lunch buddies, take turns finding healthy offerings at nearby restaurants or making something to share, and make your lunch pals walking partners if you can. There's plenty of evidence to show that people who eat nutritious lunches and take breaks actually get more work done than those who sit at their desks wolfing down a greasy fast-food lunch that will make them feel sluggish later on.

When you're home during the day, go out and walk around, take your dog for a midday stroll, or work in the yard for a few minutes—anything, just get up and move. One of my personal "desk rules" is that every time my dogs come in to ask for attention (several times a day, but not constantly), I get up and pet them or get on the floor to play for a few minutes. Often, it's just the reminder I need to get up and move around.

Doing That Thing You Do

Create one-of-a-kind individual Mini-Workouts around your personal likes, habits, interests, and idiosyncrasies. You can pretend to be a ballerina and any handy counter becomes your barre; work on whatever moves you need to become a great soccer player so you'll be ready for the next World Cup (perhaps Pelé, Marta, Mia, Beckham, or Ronaldo will be watching?); imagine you have an opportunity to practice with Cirque du Soleil in a month and really concentrate on arm exercises.

Keep It Simple and Repeatable

Whatever routine you invent, keep it simple enough that you can repeat it numerous times a day and, preferably, make it a series of moves that work your body from head to toe.

If you make it fun for yourself to get in shape (or at least kind of fun), it's more likely you'll stick with it, but if you can't make it fun, do it anyway. Before you know it, you'll see and feel real improvement and that will help keep you motivated to stick with it better than anything else.

To remind herself to keep up with her Mini-Workouts, one friend came up with the idea to post sticky notes around the house with ideas for what to do...no more forgetting!

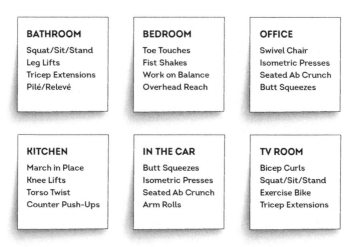

BATHROOM
Squat/Sit/Stand
Leg Lifts
Tricep Extensions
Pilé/Relevé

BEDROOM
Toe Touches
Fist Shakes
Work on Balance
Overhead Reach

OFFICE
Swivel Chair
Isometric Presses
Seated Ab Crunch
Butt Squeezes

KITCHEN
March in Place
Knee Lifts
Torso Twist
Counter Push-Ups

IN THE CAR
Butt Squeezes
Isometric Presses
Seated Ab Crunch
Arm Rolls

TV ROOM
Bicep Curls
Squat/Sit/Stand
Exercise Bike
Tricep Extensions

TURNING INTERMITTENT ACTIVITIES INTO TIME WELL SPENT

Because the activities listed above are things that almost everyone does regularly and repeatedly, it's fairly easy to link Mini-Workouts to these specific activities so that they quickly become ingrained habits. For example, while waiting for the microwave, you could do one or two sets of 16 toe touches, 16 side-step-slides, and 16 overhead arm reaches: bam, done; next time you're waiting for the microwave, same thing.

What's a little more challenging is to create routines that you can remember to link to activities that occur less frequently. You probably don't stand in line at the exact same store on a daily basis, but unless you have staff to run all your errands and do all your shopping, I guarantee the two minutes here or the five minutes there waiting in various places add up to a lot of time each week that could be put to better use than just shuffling along waiting your turn. So, while it may be a little harder to create a prompt-response link in your brain, with a bit of forethought you can find a specific stimulus to trigger your "get moving" response.

Most people frequent the same few stores every week, so when doing your regular shopping, you can use the "Express Line" sign or the bundle of helium balloons or the magazines at the checkout stand as a prompt: you see it, you move. If you regularly go to the same mall, you can plant the image in your head that as soon as you see the sign for a particular store, you'll do two or three dozen butt squeezes or make it a habit to do bicep curls as soon as you've parked the car.

Other situations may be recurring but infrequent, like taking a trip or going to a theater, concert, or sporting event, but since these kinds of activities typically necessitate long periods of sitting, it's worth your while to have some kind of (unobtrusive) Mini-Workout you can do in order to keep your muscles from getting stiff, and/or to counterbalance the excessive calories you may be consuming at a special event.

Even when a situation is completely out of the ordinary, you can always find something to serve as a prompt if you plan ahead, like wearing a special watch so whenever you check the time you think about moving. No special watch? How about putting your regular watch on the other wrist? No watch? Tie a piece of string around your finger, put a small charm on your purse handle, or put a brightly colored sticker on your cell phone so that every time you look at it, the sticker reminds you to get moving.

Look for opportunities to get up and move, even if only briefly. It may require a little creativity and discipline, but the extra minutes (or hours) of increased blood flow and improved muscle tone and balance you can achieve are worth some effort.

At the Mall

Park some distance from the mall entrance and walk around at a good clip to window shop before you get down to business. Use the stairs instead of an escalator to change levels (or walk up/down the escalator), walk back to your car to deposit packages, and plan ahead for a healthy meal strategy (sushi instead of a burger or yogurt instead of a cookie or cinnamon bun). If you live in an area with severe weather where it's impossible to spend much time outdoors at certain times of year, check your local mall to see if there are off-hours walking clubs; if the main doors open before the stores do (usually the case), you can stop by for a walk on your way to work.

I've known people who beat terrible commutes by getting up early, driving to a mall close to their workplace, taking a few laps around each floor (some malls actually have organized walking clubs), then going out for coffee or breakfast. This is a great way to start the day that leaves you feeling energized, virtuous, and ready to tackle whatever comes your way (and if you get ahead of rush hour, it minimizes time spent idling in traffic, so you use less gas). If you can find a coworker or two to meet you at the mall and join in your morning walk, so much the better, as you'll help keep each other motivated.

Standing in Line

You can turn this forced inactivity into useful time by doing subtle movements: stand on one leg, raise up on your toes repeatedly, tap your toes, trace small circles on the floor with your toes, step side-to-side, or do some simple isometric exercises like pressing your palms together.

Running Errands

When reasonable, walk from one store to the next rather than getting back in the car, but if you have to drive, at least park a little distance from the entrance—you'd be surprised how those extra steps add up. When you're on foot waiting at a traffic light, do step aerobics moves if there's a safe curb and do any of the movements mentioned above for standing in line. If there's no curb or too much traffic, just walk back and forth or, at the very least, do some butt squeezes. If you can ride your bike instead of driving, do it and invest in a basket or some panniers to hold packages or a briefcase if that will make a difference.

On an Airplane

Depending on your seat, planes can be even more constrained than cars, but the longer the flight, the more important it is to move around. You can do small versions of the seated exercises and little arm/hand/shoulder moves. On bigger planes or longer flights, you can walk up and down the aisle periodically and there is usually a space by the galley where you can do many freestanding exercises; just don't do these in front of the cockpit if you don't want to be taken for a lunatic or terrorist. If you Google "exercise on airplane," you'll find several websites that show easy exercises that won't irritate your seatmates or the flight attendants, including a pretty good site by Boeing Airlines, which inexplicably has a cartoon Cyclops demonstrating them (weird, but admittedly memorable).

Playing or Watching Sports

In reality, many people who play sports do an awful lot of standing around or, worse, sitting around (waiting your turn, getting sidelined, waiting for an opponent to do something). Stay on your feet and keep moving and walk around if possible or just step side-to-side. As for going to sporting events, for a lot of people this is even worse than sitting at home watching TV because it becomes an excuse to drink a lot of beer or eat ultra-fatty glob-snacks, and once you get into a stadium seat, it's usually really tough to get out. Walk around, get up, cheer, wave, and when snack time rolls around, be the one who offers to go get stuff and make sure you're getting something reasonable to eat like peanuts in the shell or popcorn without yellow-colored oil (stadium "butter"). Ballparks, along with most other public venues, have really improved the quality of the food they offer, so choose the good stuff and avoid the diet bombs even if other people are indulging. Ix-nay on the nachos with fake cheese.

Housecleaning

Serious housecleaning is a fair amount of exercise (scrubbing, vacuuming, mopping), but you can kick up the benefits—and dare I say, enjoyment—by putting on salsa music or rock 'n roll and having your own dance party. If you prefer classical, play something robust like the *1812 Overture* by Tchaikovsky (and I defy you to sit still when listening to the overture from Rossini's *William Tell*) and conduct the orchestra while you clean. You can also increase benefits by deliberately moving with grace and energy; instead of just picking something off the floor, pick it up by doing a toe touch and then rolling up one vertebra at a time—be creative. If you think cleaning chores have to be dull, watch Michael "Boogaloo Shrimp" Chambers taking a broom to the sidewalk in *Breakin'* or look at what Gene Kelly does with a mop in *Thousands Cheer*.

A great idea, if you can coordinate schedules, is to find a "house-cleaning buddy" with whom you share chores. It can be an hour or two at your place then on to theirs, or you can alternate weeks; an added benefit is that many tasks (like changing sheets or moving furniture so you can clean behind it) are so much easier when done by two. This can also be a good opportunity to plan a special and nutritious lunch if you make a "healthy food challenge" out of it, and alternate shopping and prep, or go out for a healthy meal as a reward for your efforts. If you can make this labor-exchange work, you and your pal can take a walk together before or after chore time and/or do something fun like ride your bikes to a nearby coffee shop.

Miscellaneous Chores

When it comes to the ordinary chores and activities that make up so much of daily life (sorting mail, washing dishes, doing laundry, taking out the trash, feeding the cat, fixing meals, making the bed, cutting the grass, setting the table), let toe-tapping can't-sit-still dance music be the soundtrack of your life and move to the beat. Make a personal party out of intermittent but recurring activities; for example, if you work on your car on the weekends, do a great job of washing and waxing it by imitating the wax-on/wax-off moves from *The Karate Kid* while listening to "You're the Best." Give yourself permission to love your life and have some fun moving around every day.

Volunteering

It may seem odd to list "volunteering" as something that will enhance your physical well-being, but studies show that people who do volunteer work have better health and report higher levels of happiness—and significantly less stress—than people who don't. When you connect with the right organization, the benefits can be fantastic, ranging from finding new friends with whom you share common interests, to providing you with professional networks to advance your career. Volunteering gives you the opportunity to share your knowledge and/or learn a new skill, helps combat loneliness, can help you overcome shyness, and can provide a sense of purpose and connection to your community. One of the great things about volunteering is that as you work to fulfill the mission of an organization you care about, it gets you out of the house and moving…sometimes so much so that it can count toward your weekly exercise total, assuming it's a regular gig. If you want to do something that really gets you in gear, think about walking dogs for the animal shelter, teaching kids to ride horses, doing trail maintenance at a local park, giving guided tours at a museum or botanical garden, or participating in the annual New Year's Day national bird count. If those seem too physically challenging, there are other kinds of activities that are less strenuous, but still get you out and moving in a positive way, like reading stories to kids at the library or helping out at a soup kitchen. Whatever gets you excited, whatever your interest may be, I guarantee there's an organization that will value the help you can provide, and you'll benefit personally in numerous ways.

> *Start where you are, use what you*
> *have, do what you can.*
>
> —Arthur Ashe
>
> American Presidential
> Medal of Freedom winner,
> three-time Grand Slam winner,
> and compassionate humanitarian

CHAPTER 5

The Movements

This is not an exercise manual per se, but rather a guide to help you get going with Mini-Workouts, plus recommendations for scheduling other exercise. If you need more direction, there are videos, books, websites, etc., with far more detail. Those new to exercise will benefit from taking a class or working with a pro to get started.

If you are able, make sure your routines include what many consider to be the absolute best exercise in the world: the squat/sit/stand. This one move strengthens thighs and butt, works abs and all the muscles that stabilize the core, and even works arms and shoulders a bit;

squat/sit/stands will build lower-body strength and rev up your metabolism faster than any other single movement. The reason I don't just use the word "squat" is because apparently many people do squats with improper form and end up injuring their knees or back (knees should never go past toes), and nothing derails fitness faster than an injury. However, everyone knows how to sit down and then stand up correctly. You can lower and lift yourself using legs only (with arms akimbo) or you can put your hands on your thighs or the arms of a chair for a boost as you stand (you'll still get tremendous benefit and won't hurt yourself).

Take 30–60 seconds to do a set every time you go to the bathroom and keep increasing the numbers as you get stronger; a toilet with a closed lid or a dining or desk chair (no wheels) is a perfect height for most people. Look for random opportunities to squat/sit/stand like during ads on TV, when on hold on the phone, when you need a break from your computer—anywhere and anytime you can, and the more the better. In addition to daily visits to the loo, identify recurring events and make them a trigger to do a set, like the arrival of the mail or hearing a nearby siren at a certain time every day; any regular occurrence in your environment can serve as a prompt. A set for you may be three or ten or thirty; you want to do enough that you feel you're making an effort, but not like you're going to pass out.

You may decide on "quick sets" of, say, five or 10 that you do most of the time, but then once or twice a day you do 15 or 30 or 50. Figure out the right number for your current fitness level and then get moving. In a world of gadgets and increasing complication, this sounds way too simple, but take these words at face value; they are not secret code. To be clear: "squat" means stick your butt out as you bend your knees; "sit" means put your backside down on a chair, bench, or closed toilet seat; "stand" means stand up; "repeat" means do it again. Try it—this one move can work miracles. Seriously—it's amazing.

I'm describing many different exercises to give you options for designing Mini-Workouts that you like, but choose only a few to work into routines to perform repeatedly. If you get bored, come back to the list for more ideas or just make up a routine for yourself. I've tried to describe movements clearly, but if you don't understand my directions, just choose something else or improvise. There are numerous books, websites, DVDs, and YouTube videos demonstrating various exercises, but be advised that quality is all over the map, so be discriminating. Simple movements like sitting down and standing up are so straightforward you needn't worry about form, but if you want to work with weights or try something more complicated where there's potential for injury, you'd probably benefit from some professional instruction, especially if you're new to exercising. Most health clubs offer free trials and every community has free or inexpensive classes through the local recreation department, community or senior center, or a local pro may organize casual group meetups at a nearby park (check social media or the library bulletin board). If you can afford it, hiring a personal trainer can be a worthwhile investment to get you started and/or keep you motivated.

SIMPLE EXERCISES YOU CAN DO EVERY DAY

The following movements need no special equipment and can be done with or without support depending on space, and whether or not you have good balance. Be creative, this is just a sampling.

Arm and Shoulder Exercises

- Overhead arm reaches—one at a time or both together, arms reach straight up like you're pushing something up onto a high shelf or reaching for a star

- Overhead reach/pull down—the reverse of
  the overhead reach so the effort comes on the
  downward motion, making a fist as you slowly pull
  down (on an imaginary rope)

- Overhead arm reaches with a side stretch—alternate
  reaching up then over your head and out to the side;
  this works often-ignored side muscles (obliques)

- Front bicep curls—with arms straight out in front
  (either one at a time or both together) alternate
  quick movements with slow motion curls; change
  hand position for variation

- Tricep extensions—bend arms so fists are close
  to shoulders; with arms tight to your sides, slowly
  straighten, then raise hands up in back; lean
  forward a little

- Side arm pushes with a torso twist—keep hand flat
  as you push away, twisting from side-to-side (right
  hand pushes past left side/left past right)

- Wax on/wax off—like in *The Karate Kid*, circular
  movements as if you're applying then removing
  car wax

- Front arm rolls—with elbows bent, hold both arms
  up in front (like in *I Dream of Jeannie* as she casts

her spell) then roll one hand over the other to the front, then reverse

- Side arm circles—with arms held straight out to the side, make circles forward then back, both small and large, palms up then palms down

- The queen's wave—bent elbows with arms held parallel out in front, rotate your hands

- Prayer position lifts—with hands together and elbows close together or touching, raise hands up and down

- Prayer position open and close—start with hands in the same position as above, then bring your elbows back as far as you can (the classic western movie response to "put 'em up!"), then back together again in front

- Put 'em up lifts—with arms at sides, raise hands up and down

- Chicken wing flaps—with hands at armpits, flap elbows straight up and down

- Isometric presses—push hands against one another

- Swimming arm moves—breaststroke, front crawl, backstroke

- Shake, shake, shake—both hands together or one at a time, rapid moves like shaking dice, castanets, or a martini shaker

Seated Exercises for
Legs/Butt/Feet/Abdominals/Core

- With knees bent, lift one leg at a time up off the floor—be sure to tighten your core as you do this (you can lift higher as you get stronger)

- Lift legs off the floor separately, flex your feet, then make foot-ankle circles with a pointed toe

- Leg lift crunch—sit up straight and tighten everything while slowly lifting both legs up together with knees bent, then slowly lower

- Alternate heel and toe raises—start with feet flat on the floor and slowly raise toes, back to flat, then raise heels

- Toe taps front and side-to-side—heel stays in place as ankle swivels

- Butt squeezes—imagine there's a check for a million dollars between your sweet cheeks that you'll lose if you don't hold tight

- If seated in a swivel chair, swivel back and forth while facing forward and keeping your shoulders parallel to the desk

- Abdominal workout—sit with hips well back in the chair and hands in your lap or behind your head, lean forward and upright, then slowly sit back until touching the back of the chair

- Seated abdominal crunches—sitting with feet flat and knees apart, slowly sit forward and put hands on the floor and then slowly straighten up (provides a nice stretch for back and shoulders at the same time)

Freestanding Leg Exercises

- March in place
- Leg-lifts with a flexed foot straight up to the side, down, out to the back corner, down, then straight back
- Leg-lifts as above but with toes pointed
- First position plié—bend knees with heels touching and heels pointed out, straighten up, go up your toes (relevé), repeat

- Second position plié—bend knees, feet shoulder width apart and toes pointed out, plié then relevé (down then up)

- Trace circles on the floor with your toes, in front then in back

- Knee lift—one leg lifts repeatedly with arms out for balance and abdominals tight (hold onto something if necessary)

- Celtic dance heel-toe taps—tap heel in front, toe tap in front of opposite foot, heel tap again, change sides

Full Body Movements

- Celtic dance heel-toe taps stepping side-to-side and with a little jump if you have room and inclination

- Practice sports moves (do both sides): air-dribbling, tennis serve, swing a baseball bat or golf club (real or pretend), shoot baskets; imagination and the space available are your only limits

- March in place with arms swinging vigorously

- Jog in place

- Step to the side then slide/drag the other foot over to touch heels, then back the other way

- Hip wiggles from side-to-side (think hula)

- Pelvic tilts (think sex)

- Grapevine step—sidestep right behind left for three or more steps, then back the other way left behind right, repeat crossing over in front

- Bounce a ball (real or pretend)

- Step-aerobic moves—step up/down repeatedly using any stair-step or aerobic step equipment (take a class or get a book for variations)

- Toe touches—feet shoulder width apart, bend straight down to touch your toes, slowly straighten up (if you can't reach your toes, go to your knees); then touch your toes with the opposite hand (right hand to left foot/left hand to right foot)

- Toe touches with a twist—as above, but touch hand to opposite foot or knee, then reach hands up (like making the "Y" for the song "YMCA")

- Swimmers' arms—breaststroke, front crawl, and backstroke—you can do leg moves at the same time if you're sufficiently coordinated

- Windmill arms front and back—either slowly or moderately quickly, windmill your arms to your fullest range of motion (the highest, biggest circle you can make)

- Any dance: salsa, the twist, cha-cha-cha, the Watusi, Macarena, moonwalk, disco, the funky chicken, waltz, polka, Charleston, the bump, pogo, punk-funk, line dances, can-can, the hustle, and let's not forget the YMCA or any ballet moves you may know

- Skip, hop, jump!

Stretching/Loosening Movements

For maximum benefit, hold the following stretches for 15–30 seconds; these moves should all be done v-e-r-r-r-y s-l-o-w-l-y.

- Shoulder rolls front and back—make circles with your shoulders (up, around, down)

- Shoulder shrugs—bring shoulders straight up toward ears, then straight down

- Hand flexes—spread fingers to the max, then make a fist

- Hand/arm stretches—with fingers interlaced, press arms out straight with palms out and hold the stretch, then lift straight up overhead and hold

- Chest stretch—after doing the above, bring hands down behind your head and press elbows back

- Wrist rolls—hold arms straight out in front and roll your hands and wrists in and out

- Ankle rolls—make a circle with your toe pointed

- Hugs—give yourself a big hug, getting your hands as far around your back as possible

- Neck stretch—leading with your chin, look as far over your shoulder as you can and hold, then to the other side

- Corner neck stretch—point your nose toward your armpit and drop your chin (for a more intense stretch, put your hand on your head)

- Runners' stride—one knee bent, other leg with heel flat on the floor behind you and feet pointed straight front (best done holding onto wall or counter, and don't let front knee extend past front toes)

- Calf and foot stretch—toes up against a wall and lean into it

- Stair calf stretch—while standing on a step where you can hold securely to the railing, keep one foot flat and secure on the step and drop the other heel off the edge

- Toe touches—bend over to touch toes, hold for a moment to stretch your back then slowly roll up one vertebra at a time

- Yoga stretching movements (take a class or get a video if you're a beginner)

Floor Exercises

- Bent knee sit-ups (don't strain your neck, your core should be doing the work)

- Pelvic lifts—lying flat with knees bent and arms at your sides, lift hips up off the floor (squeeze your butt) either quickly or slowly (up/squeeze/down/relax/up squeeze…etc.)

- Bridge lifts—as above, but bring your hips up to where they form a straight line from knees to shoulders and hold the position

- Crisscross front and back—with legs straight up in the air, legs go out to form a V then back together, crossing one foot over the other

- Bicycle and reverse bicycle—with back flat on floor and legs up, ride an imaginary bike leading with your heels

- Heels to ceiling—with legs up but knees bent, straighten legs with heel pointing toward ceiling, slowly bend and repeat

- Side twist stretches—with back flat on floor, knees up but bent and tight together, drop both legs over to one side (use your hands for support and keep shoulders more or less flat); hold, come back to center, then slowly lower to the other side

- Yoga floor exercises—if you're new to yoga, take a class for beginners or watch a video by an experienced pro

Great! Fantastic! You've now got some Mini-Workout routines to start turning into habits, so no matter what else is going on in your life, make time to give yourself a big hug several times a day and hold it for a moment or two to stretch out your neck, shoulders, and back, as you congratulate yourself for consistently doing a little bit here and a little bit there to improve your health. Smile at yourself often to reaffirm that you like yourself and deserve to be cared for. The very act of smiling will reduce stress levels and boost your mood and self-esteem…so go ahead and feel pleased with yourself, you deserve it.

Love yourself; that's the single most powerful thing.

Out of that springs:

How are you eating?
How are you exercising?
How are you resting?

—Nia Peeples

American Heart
Association spokesperson,
actress, singer, dancer, and
health and fitness writer

CHAPTER 6

Mini-Workouts: Adding It All Up

You may ask, "Can Mini-Workouts really make a difference?" It may surprise you to see how quickly consistent daily repetitions can add up to an impressive number, and how enough tiny blocks of time here and there can turn into a meaningful number of minutes (or even hours) over the course of a week. The following is just one example.

Let's say you have an electric toothbrush that goes in 30-second cycles. That's one cycle for each quadrant of your mouth, so four cycles total, plus many dentists recommend two more cycles for good measure. That means three minutes of brushing at night and another three in the morning. While brushing, you can do any combination of standing leg exercises; one easy routine would be leg lifts to the side, the back corner, and then straight back. If you haven't exercised in a while, maybe you can only do one leg lift every five seconds, but if you're in somewhat decent shape you may be able to average one per second. So, just standing at the sink (which you do anyway), over the course of a week, without breaking a sweat, putting on shoes, or going anywhere...

> 1 leg lift every 5 seconds for 6 minutes
> = 42 minutes per week of exercising
>> = 72 leg lifts per day x 7 days
>> = 504 leg lifts per week

> 1 leg lift every 1 second for 6 minutes
> = 42 minutes per week of exercising
>> = 360 leg lifts per day x 7 days
>> = 2520 leg lifts per week

Maybe you think doing 72 or 360 leg lifts in a day would be impossible and you can't imagine devoting 42 minutes a week just to doing leg lifts, but when you're counting off the seconds as you brush your teeth, it's just 30 side...30 corner...30 back / change sides / 30 side...30 corner...30 back and zip! zip! zip! teeth are clean, gluteus maximus is worked. Even at only one every five seconds (or if you don't brush for a full three minutes), the number is enough that you can see how a little persistence can pay off very quickly in terms of a tighter, stronger bum—better in the jeans and easier to climb stairs.

MEASURING TIME AND COUNTING REPETITIONS

What is more important, the number of minutes spent exercising or the number of reps you do? Like so many things in life, the answer is: it depends. In the case of Mini-Workouts, the time spent doing them is important only in a very general way; what matters is that you work your muscles and boost your metabolism numerous times every day so that over the course of the week you're improving your overall fitness. The amount of time spent, the speed at which you move, and the number of repetitions you do will be determined by your personal ability and motivation. On a typical day you may do lots and lots of quick Mini-Workouts ranging from 15–90 seconds each and then several longer routines that take two to five minutes. You may not know or care how long any of these activities take individually, but if you're curious (especially if you like to measure things), it might be interesting to keep track for a few days to see what your average time adds up to.

With some Mini-Workout routines, like the electric toothbrush example given above, it's easy to calculate time since the number of minutes is always the same, but most people are likely to find keeping a running total of other movements difficult and tedious (e.g., 30 seconds + 60 + 20 + 90 + 15 + 60 + 45 + 150 + 30 + 20 + 90 + etcetera). However, if you're curious to see how many minutes you spend doing Mini-Workouts, go ahead and track them, because setting and achieving a specific time target just might be the thing that helps keep you motivated all week. The important thing about Mini-Workouts is that you establish routines—and stick to them—and continue to challenge yourself by upping the number of reps you do in a set and looking for opportunities to move more, like taking the stairs instead of an escalator or parking farther from the entrance to a store.

There are also other kinds of exercise, such as lifting weights or using resistance bands, where the number of repetitions or the amount of effort are the important factors, rather than the amount of time spent doing them. If you're using handweights that are close to the maximum you can manage, it would take a lot of effort to do 10 bicep curls, but it would sound like you'd done nothing if you said you'd exercised for less than a minute, whereas you might have actually increased your strength and stamina in a very meaningful way.

On the other hand, when it comes to aerobic exercise, time matters very much indeed. The US Department of Health and Human Services recommends a minimum of 150 minutes of moderate activity or 75 minutes of vigorous activity per week to keep your heart in good condition, so you must make sure that whatever walking and exercise schedule you establish gets you to at least that minimum… after you surpass the minimum, whether or not you count and tally the extra time is up to you. Personally, I usually take a one-hour water aerobics class once or twice a week (if there's no pandemic) and I walk my dogs numerous times during the week and march in place when they stop to sniff something interesting (rain or shine, they've gotta go). So even though I have only a vague idea of how many minutes of aerobic exercise I do every week, I know I'm well beyond the minimum and I'm not inclined to keep track of the rest because that's not the way my brain works. When I'm trying to lose some weight, even though I don't set a specific time target, I make a point of adding a little extra time to my classes and possibly add an extra class to the week's schedule, and I take a longer route when I walk the dogs and give them a nice surprise. Other people prefer to calculate their activities with much more precision and many people get a great sense of satisfaction from keeping a detailed journal or logbook (keeping a journal has been shown to be an effective motivator for people who keep up with it). A friend and I occasionally meet at the pool and then go out for coffee afterward. When I do laps on my own, I swim for approximately a half hour (could be 27 minutes, could be 33, depending on my mood), but when I meet my friend, we swim for exactly 30 minutes because she sets the timer on her watch when we start and the second the alarm goes off, she stops. Although we both keep moving the whole time, she knows exactly how many laps she swam, what her average speed was, which lap was her fastest, and whether or not she met or exceeded her usual pace; I, on the other hand, just know that I did laps for half an hour. My friend is an accountant and she derives great satisfaction from counting and measuring; I am a writer and a cook and like to use my pool time thinking about recipes or articles or just daydreaming.

With all of this in mind, figure out what approach works best for you and is sustainable. In the calculations below, I've listed minutes in places where it's easy to measure the time, but for many of your Mini-Workouts, you'll need to count for yourself if you want to know the total number of minutes you're putting in, since speed and effort will vary from person to person. One easy way would be to just count how many minutes of Mini-Workout time is spent in each location, rather than on individual moves. For example, you could figure your total in the bedroom was three minutes followed by four minutes in the kitchen, and so on throughout the day.

DAILY / WEEKLY / MONTHLY
CALCULATIONS

Let's do a calculation that assumes a fairly modest level of effort over the course of a single day and see what that adds up to in a week and for a 30-day month...assuming you really do your Mini-Workouts every day. The following is a sample of routines chosen randomly. When you look at the repetition totals you can see that even if you were to do only a quarter of this number, all these little things can add up quickly and make an impressive difference.

Though your personal numbers will vary, time totals are given in the hypothetical examples below that demonstrate how much time is typically spent every day doing practically nothing while you wait for something to happen and/or are stuck in a seat somewhere (desk, car, plane, theater, stadium). With a small amount of effort, that time can instead be used to improve your strength, flexibility, balance, and coordination. Having mini-goals for your Mini-Workouts can relieve tedium and boredom as well; for example, if there's an intersection where you get stuck every day while commuting, instead of being bored or aggravated, you can think of it as an opportunity to do a Mini-Workout routine and even come up with specific playlists to listen to in the car that make you want to move.

Daily Routines in the Bathroom

Teeth brushing, flossing, and other ablutions 2x/day = 6 minutes total

> 1 leg lift every 3 sec = 20 per min
>> [total 120]

Waiting for water to get hot/washing & drying hands/ using lotion = 6 minutes total

Overhead reaches left & right 25 per min
(2x/day = 2 min)
[total 50]

Knee lifts 10 per side per min
(2x/day 30 sec each = 1 min)
[total 20]

Triceps extensions both arms 25 per min
(2x/day = 2 min)
[total 50]

Plié (bend knees) then revelé (up on toes) 40 per min
(2x/day 30 sec each = 1 min)
[total 40]

Using the bathroom 6x/day (time not calculated and please don't tell me how long you're in there)

Biceps curls 15 each bathroom visit
[total 90]

Prayer position arms open/close 5 each
bathroom visit
[total 30]

Squat/sit/stands 1 set of 10 each visit
[total 60]

Total Time—12 minutes (plus however many minutes you spend doing arm movements while taking care of business and doing squat/sit/stands afterward)

Daily Routines in the Kitchen

Waiting for the microwave/sink tap/coffee pot/toaster,
3 min 5x day = 15 min total

Marching in place (knees high) 30 steps per min
(2x/day = 2 min)
[total 60]

Overhead reaches left & right 25 per min
(2x/day = 2 min)
[total 50]

One leg lift every 3 seconds = 20 per min
(5x/day = 5 min)
[total 100]

Torso twist arm presses left & right 20 per min
(2x/day = 2 min)
[total 40]

Second position plié/relevé 20 per min
(2x/day 30 sec = 1 min)
[total 20]

Hula hip wiggles 40 per min
(2x/day 30 sec each = 1 min)
[total 40]

Front arm rolls 100 per min
(2x/day 30 sec each = 1 min)
[total 100]

Reverse arm rolls 100 per min
(2x/day 30 sec each = 1 min)
[total 100]

Total Time—30 minutes

Daily Routines while Commuting
(Car, Bus, Subway, Train, or Ferry)

Using the time spent getting from point A to point B; though most commutes are far longer, I'm estimating a mere four minutes each way being put to use; if you're alone or if your whole carpool group is onboard with this program, you can do much more.

Butt squeezes 20 per min
(2x/day = 2 min)
[total 40]

Toe taps 60 per min
(2x/day 1 min each = 2 min)
[total 120]

Isometric arm presses (press/hold/release every
2 secs = 30/min)
(4x/day 30 sec each = 2 min)
[total 60]

Seated abdominal crunches 20 per min
(2x/day = 2 min)
[total 40]

Total Time—8 minutes

Daily Office Routines

Putting wasted time to good use and intentionally interrupting periods of sedentary inactivity, 10 minutes per day

Seated abdominal crunches, 10 every 30 secs
  (4x/day = 2 min)
  [total 40]

Squat/sit/stands, 10 every 30 secs
  (4x/day = 2 min)
  [total 40]

Overhead reaches, 10 on each side
  (4x/day = 4 min)
  [total 40]

Butt squeezes, 20 per min
  (2x/day = 2 min)
  [total 40]

Total Time—20 minutes

SAMPLE COMPILATION

The following chart demonstrates the number of repetitions that can be accomplished in a 30-day month by consistently doing daily Mini-Workouts. You'll eventually figure out what routines suit you best, but this random selection of moves would work every major pair of muscles in the body. The exact amount of time will depend on your personal ability and the moves you decide on, but for purposes of this hypothetical example, let's assume one second for each of the movements listed.

Movement	Daily	Weekly	Monthly
Squat/sit/stands	100	700	3,000
Leg lifts	120	840	3,600
Bicep curls	90	630	2,700
Prayer position (open/close)	30	210	900
Overhead reaches	200	1,400	6,000
Knee lifts	10	70	300
Tricep extensions	50	350	1,500
Plié, then relevé	40	280	1,200
March in place	60	420	1,800

Movement	Daily	Weekly	Monthly
Torso twist pushes	40	280	1,200
Second position plié/relevé	20	140	600
Hula hip wiggles	40	280	1,200
Front arm rolls	100	700	3,000
Reverse arm rolls	100	700	3,000
Butt squeezes	80	560	2,400
Toe taps	120	840	3,600
Isometric arm presses	60	420	1,800
Seated abdominal crunches	40	280	1,200
TOTAL SECONDS **TOTAL MINUTES** **TOTAL HOURS**	1,300 22 .36	9,100 151 2.5	39,000 645.6 10.76

Look how these add up! And this tally doesn't even count all the other random beneficial things you can do like taking the stairs instead of using the elevator, toe-tapping at the grocery store or anywhere else you have to wait, and taking advantage of appropriate situations (sporting events, conferences, parties, rallies, parades, etc.) to stay on your feet and walk around rather than sitting still for an extended period of time. All you're doing is turning formerly wasted standing- or sitting-around time into productive help-your-body time.

When you look at the total number of repetitions, you might think "Impossible! I could never do that many," but when you think about doing five here and 10 or 20 there, you realize, "Well, sure...I can do that." Once a Mini-Workout is inextricably linked with an activity, it's almost harder *not* to do it than to do it because good habits are nearly as difficult to break as bad ones. If you add Mini-Workouts to your daily schedule (assuming you're doing some walking and/or other aerobic activity), you've got a movement routine that will keep your brain and vital organs functioning well for life. You'll feel more energized, have more stamina to meet the demands of the day, and more resilience for when a virus crosses your path. If and when you decide you want to move to a higher fitness level, just add more time to this regimen, up the amount of time spent walking, add an aerobics class, increase the intensity of your workouts, and/or move up to slightly heavier hand weights (see Muscle Strength in the next chapter).

You can start figuring out right now—right this minute—what Mini-Workouts you like and which of your daily activities you can easily link them to. If you read a lot, for example, you might decide that whenever you get to the end of a section or chapter, you'll stop reading and do a set of squat/sit/stands. Here we are at the end of this section, so:

Stop reading now and ... Squat ... Sit ... Stand ...

Squat ... Sit ... Stand ... Squat ... Sit ... Go!!!

ARE DAILY MINI-WORKOUT ROUTINES YOUR NEW NORMAL?

If so, CONGRATULATIONS & HURRAH!!! Go ahead and give yourself a big pat on the back, because you've successfully turned Mini-Workouts into part of your regular routine...at least, I hope you have, or soon will. Once you realize how easy it is to reap great rewards from Mini-Workouts without totally disrupting your regular schedule—and that those rewards are amazing compared with the small effort required—and you steadily get stronger and feel noticeably better as a result, chances are good you will soon want to learn about the benefits that can be derived from other kinds of exercise.

Are You Ready to Think about Moving More?

- You've been doing MINI-WORKOUTS every day and are now noticeably less flabby than before and well on the way to being in control of your health.

- Incorporating a WALKING PROGRAM into your schedule will bring tremendous benefits to both appearance and health, from head to toe, inside and out.

- The more you walk, the more energy and stamina you will have as you strengthen muscles, bones, and joints, and rev up your metabolism.

- You can start slowly and increase gradually until walking becomes an enjoyable part of your regular routine.

- Some of you may even want to start playing a sport or try a new exercise class, or decide it would be rewarding to join a fitness center or gym.

If you're ready to spend more time exercising, in the next chapter we'll ask and answer some important questions about human bodies and what they need; however—and this is an important "however"—if you feel like you're simply not up to making any more changes right now, just put this book aside and come back to it when you're ready to take the next step. Don't feel pressured into making changes faster than you can incorporate them, because feeling overwhelmed will probably send you to the couch feeling depressed, with a mountain of junk food to snarf down. Improvement will come inch-by-inch, step-by-step, poco-a-poco, bit-by-bit as you progressively move toward a healthier future self.

> *Enlightenment must come little-by-little, otherwise it would overwhelm.*
>
> —Idries Shah
>
> Afghan-Indian Sufi author, scholar, teacher, and publisher

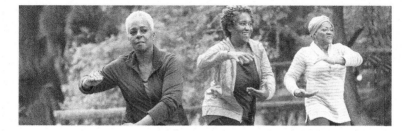

CHAPTER 7

What Exercising Does for Your Body

While you may not have any particular interest in playing sports or being super active, you undoubtedly want to feel well, sleep well, avoid illness as much as possible, and have enough energy and strength for life's normal activities. It would also be nice to have sufficient stamina to meet the occasional demand like sprinting to catch a plane or running after a wayward puppy or child without collapsing, right?

What can you do to achieve these goals?

- Do Mini-Workouts throughout the day, every day
- Aim to walk two and a half hours per week (divide in increments to suit your schedule, various options are listed below)
- Stretch for two or three minutes after your walks
- Take a few slow deep breaths after exercising, before going to bed, or any time you need to relax
- Work on balance two minutes twice a week and a few moments here and there
- Use hand weights or stretch bands a few minutes two or three times a week to build muscle

That's not really so onerous, is it? And before you start complaining that you're too busy to walk 30 minutes five times a week (or 15 minutes 10 times a week), take a look at how much time you spend watching TV, surfing the web, texting friends, shopping online, watching cat videos, looking at social media, reading ten versions of the same news story, tweeting, flipping through magazines, watching sports, playing word games, etc., and tell me you can't cut back on one or two of these activities enough to enjoy the benefits of a good night's sleep, less time spent being sick, having fewer aches and pains, having more energy, and potentially a longer, more enjoyable life. If you do more, you'll benefit in other ways, but if you can manage the suggestions above the majority of the time (perfection not required), you have a very good chance of enjoying a healthy life for your full allotment of years, whatever that may be.

The single *best* exercise for human health is WALKING, but the *fastest* way to see that you are getting stronger week-by-week is with MINI-WORKOUTS, so that's the best (and the easiest) place to start. In a matter of days you can increase the number of squat/sit/stands or arm circles you can do in one go, and in a matter of weeks, flab begins to be replaced by muscle definition. This rapid improvement will help keep you motivated to stay focused on your health.

As soon as you're ready—and it should be soon—it's time to begin a walking program. As your walking routine becomes easier over time, you can gradually increase the distance, pick up your pace, and walk more often. The visible benefits are more subtle than the quick results you see with Mini-Workouts, but a stronger heart and increased lung capacity are key to living a healthy life, and putting one foot in front of the other is the surest path to improvement. You may start out at a very leisurely stroll, but once you've established a comfortable routine at your current level, you can bring your speed and time up enough to get valuable aerobic benefits.

Walking at a good clip, for enough time, covering sufficient distance, and walking up and down hills (or mountains) can absolutely give you sufficient aerobic exercise to stay healthy even if you never set foot in a gym in your life; indeed, walking is the primary exercise of the many centenarians who make up the five "Blue Zones" on the planet, which are places around the world where people live unusually long healthy lives (more details under Finding Walking Partners). However, there are also many enjoyable classes and fun activities that are hard to organize on your own that are available at health clubs, exercise studios, or through your local recreation department, if you prefer to have company when you exercise. Those activities can include partner dancing, Pilates reformer, paddle tennis, martial arts, hydro-biking, fencing, dance or water aerobics, etc. Even though going to structured classes isn't required, I'm including information about the benefits of recreational sports and play, and general information on what you can get out of a health-club membership, because most people work harder with a pal or in a structured class under the guidance of a good teacher than when they're on their own.

Additionally, many people live in communities that are not very pedestrian-friendly or where the weather is less than inviting at certain times of year, so going outside to walk is not always a viable option (exercising in blizzard conditions or heat over 100° can actually kill you...not our goal). Once you start seeing improvements in your fitness and stamina, you may be motivated to start doing some of the activities that made you happy when you were younger.

While your motivation for getting in shape may be the desire to look a certain way or fit into a favorite pair of jeans that currently make you feel like a stuffed sausage, the simple fact of the matter is that you need to move to live. You have to take in oxygen and pump blood from head to toe and back again, and the only way to do that enough to be healthy is to move.

Your body is active 24/7 doing things such as digesting food, healing cuts, clearing waste, producing new cells, fighting viruses, growing nails and hair, producing tears, making an interesting variety of sounds, moving the 43 muscles of your face to express an incredible variety of emotions, replacing eyelashes, thinking about multiple things at once, producing sperm or ova, sending electrical impulses from end to end, sensing danger, lubricating joints, looking in multiple directions at the same time, sending hunger signals from the gut to the brain, flexing limbs, experiencing pain and pleasure, strengthening tendons, listening to several conversations simultaneously, blinking, forming opinions, making decisions, regulating hormones, contracting and coordinating muscles so you can move from place to place, smelling the world, sneezing, coughing, expanding and contracting the lungs, evaluating information, and at certain times of life, growing bones and teeth, starting a beard, creating a baby, or producing milk.

Whew! So, while your body is busy doing all these things behind the scenes, what are you—that is to say, the decision-making conscious part of your brain—doing to help or hinder all this hard work?

Make no mistake, there is a direct connection between movement and a healthy body and mind, and you ignore this simple fact at your peril. Let's take a look at how exercise and movement affect different parts of the body, clarify what you need to do in order to keep your brain and internal systems functioning well and your immune system at the ready, and analyze what that means in terms of health, longevity, wellness, and your overall sense of yourself.

DETAILS OF THE SIX ELEMENTS OF FITNESS

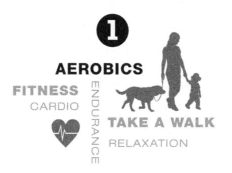

Aerobic fitness is your body's ability to take up oxygen, transfer it into the blood, and pump the blood through the heart, out to the extremities, and back again, in order to meet whatever energy demands are placed upon it. The lungs and heart are muscles that, like every other muscle in the body, can be in excellent or lousy shape depending on how they are used, not used, or misused. Fortunately, they can easily be improved even after a long period of neglect, and the best way to accomplish this is through aerobic exercise, which is defined as moderate-to-fairly intense exercise performed for an extended period of time, typically 15–90 minutes per session. Recommendations by experts for weekly totals vary, but there is a lot of consensus that two and half hours a week (150 minutes) is a reasonable amount for the average adult. This can be done with whatever activities and time sessions best suit your schedule, personality, and level of ability (make sure to add 3–5 minutes for warm-up before starting an aerobic workout in order to prevent muscle strain). Of course, if you can do more, so much the better, but don't try to do so much that you defeat yourself.

If you've been sedentary for a long time or are recovering from injury or illness, two and half hours a week may be unrealistic, but can be something to aim for. If all you can manage at one time is five minutes, then do five minutes and be proud of yourself for doing what you can. Your near- to medium-term goal can include doing two or more five-minute sessions a day and aiming for modest increases to seven, eight, or 10 minutes at a time. Don't despair if you're as weak as a newborn kitten, just meet yourself where you are right now and put one foot in front of the other both literally and figuratively.

The word "aerobic" means "with oxygen," so the goal is to exercise with enough intensity that you breathe more quickly and deeply than when at rest, but not so hard you're gasping for air. The general rule of thumb is that you should be able to carry on a conversation, but not sing. In addition to improving lung and heart strength and capacity, aerobic exercise also burns fat cells (exercise is initially fueled by carbohydrates, but after about 15 minutes the body begins to burn stored fat), strengthens the muscles of the whole body, improves circulation, lowers blood pressure, and reduces stress. It also makes you feel really good, because besides the glow you get from feeling virtuous, when moving at an aerobic pace the body releases endorphins into the bloodstream, the natural painkillers that give you a sense of well-being sometimes described as a natural high.

Aerobic activities include:

- Walking at a moderate to very brisk pace (sidewalk, trail, beach, treadmill, or track)
- Swimming laps, water aerobics, hydro-biking
- Bicycle riding outside or on a stationary bike (or spinning)
- Boxing and wrestling
- Some martial arts
- Dancing and dance-exercise (Zumba, Jazzercise, etc.)
- Jogging or speed walking
- Step aerobics
- Hooping, aka hula hooping

- Skateboarding, skating, or rollerblading
- Mowing the lawn (unless it's a riding mower)
- Stair climbing for 15+ minutes (up and down flights of stairs or stair machine)
- Digging holes and trenches or other extended garden work
- Table tennis, aka ping-pong
- Kayaking, canoeing, or sculling
- Soccer, hockey, or lacrosse
- Jumping rope
- Racquet sports where you stay on the move 15+ minutes
- Cross-country skiing
- Hiking and hill climbing
- Ice skating and ice hockey

Aerobic fitness is the only element of fitness that cannot be achieved with a Mini-Workout since, by definition, you need a sustained effort for a minimum of fifteen minutes (some experts say 10 minutes if you really exert yourself right from the first second). There are many sports that are good exercise but are not aerobic because the exertion is done in short bursts followed by inactivity; however, you can achieve aerobic benefits from some of your favorite pastimes by using what is normally down-time to walk around (somewhat vigorously) or march in place while swinging your arms. One example would be playing tennis: for most amateurs, the periods of exercise (serving, running, hitting) are interspersed with longer periods of waiting for someone to retrieve a ball or get ready to serve. To make your game aerobic (remember, 15 minutes or more of sustained activity at a high enough level that you're breathing medium-hard), you must run or walk quickly (not stroll) to get an out-of-bounds ball, and during wait periods, rapidly move back and forth, swinging your racket or marching in place. Professional tennis players typically have long periods of high-level aerobic activity interspersed with short bursts of intense all-out effort (anaerobic activity), interspersed with short breaks of rest or low-level activity for recovery, but most amateurs rarely sustain a high level of exertion for more than a few minutes at a time. However, staying on the move can easily change that. Bowling is another example of sporadic exercise followed by a whole lot of sitting. If you want to get real benefits from going bowling, stay on your feet and keep moving while waiting for your turn; you'll also get extra rewards if you keep holding, lifting, or swinging the ball in anticipation of the next strike.

Aerobic Exercise with Bursts of Anaerobic Activity

"Anaerobic" means "in the absence of oxygen" and exercises described as anaerobic are activities performed at such a high level of intensity that it's not possible to replenish oxygen in the body during the exercise. A truly all-out effort (the maximum possible energy expenditure or close to it) can only be sustained for 20–90 seconds and must be followed immediately by a period of rest/recovery (gasping and gulping in air). Trained athletes can go a little longer but note that many competitive runners literally collapse on the ground after their sprints…they go full out and then are done, done, done, and can't do one more thing (not even sit up) until they replenish spent oxygen. Unless you're in the Olympics and going for the gold, I don't recommend aiming for the 100 percent effort level, as there is always the possibility of a sprain, muscle tear, or other injury. Anaerobic exercise promotes muscle mass, strength, speed, and power, but it's best to keep your personal "all-out" effort somewhere in the 75–85 percent effort range, as an injury can put you out of commission for weeks or months—think how many pros get sidelined by injury, even with perfectly honed bodies and professional coaches—so proceed with caution.

Bursts of anaerobic activity are sometimes mixed in as part of an aerobic exercise routine and can boost weight loss as well as increasing strength, because when demand is sustained after oxygen is depleted, the body goes elsewhere for energy—namely into stored fat—and your metabolism changes. This is the principle behind the High Intensity Interval Training (HIIT) classes offered at gyms (they may call them Tabata or Plyometrics), but please note these are not for beginners, nor for people with heart disease or certain other ailments. Kids often indulge in anaerobic activities just for fun, like when they suddenly just run as fast as they possibly can or jump up and down until they drop from exhaustion. There's something very satisfying about pushing yourself to the limit (I sometimes take a water aerobics Tabata class that I simultaneously love and hate), but if you want to try a HIIT routine, do it in a supervised class with a knowledgeable instructor. If you've been exercising for a while, are in fairly decent shape, and are ready to take your routines up a notch, try adding a little HIIT to your workout. If you regularly jog or run, you can intersperse jogging with some sprints; if bike riding is your thing, include spurts of pedaling as fast as you can for 20 or 30 seconds, then recover by moving at a very slow pace for a few minutes before doing another one.

If you'd like to flirt with the principle without actually going for anything close to the maximum effort, you can incorporate short periods of slightly higher than normal effort into your regular routine. For example, if you're walking at a medium pace, every five minutes you can do one minute of very brisk walking or even break into a jog, then slow back down to your regular pace and catch your breath.

Though you can't improve aerobic fitness with Mini-Workouts, you can achieve short bursts of anaerobic level activity by rapidly doing 30–60 seconds of a routine that lends itself to smooth repetitive motion (like squat/sit/stands or marching in place with arms swinging); however, this is something to work up to and try after a month or two, not for someone just starting to get active after a long period of being sedentary.

Aerobic Exercise Trends and Fads

Styles change constantly, and what's popular one season may be forgotten—or even sneered at—the next. In every aspect of life from clothes to cuisine to tech gadgets, there are periodic fads that are a flash in the pan, updated approaches to keep old standbys fresh, changes in thinking based on new information, and, occasionally, true innovations. Exercise programs are not exempt from the vagaries of taste, and since we need to keep moving for our entire lives, it's inevitable that creative entrepreneurs will keep coming up with novel ways to make exercise programs fun for us and make a profit for themselves. Some fads, like the vibrating platform and belt, deservedly fade into oblivion, but the appeal of getting shaken into muscular perfection without having to make any effort is understandable—just think if you could be in perfect shape by standing on a box and fastening a strap around your hips. However, the human body is designed for motion and since we Americans love whatever is new, it's inevitable that the "latest thing" will continue to evolve from year to year. It's up to you to make a smart decision about how worthwhile—or not—the latest exercise program is. Here are a couple of trends I think are worth mentioning since they've been getting a lot of media attention for quite a while.

The Four-Second Workout

The upshot is that if you interrupt your normal routine of sitting on your rump for eight-to-ten hours a day with four-second bursts of intense activity, there are certain health benefits to be found.

The headline version of this story is that a four-second "workout" every hour will keep you healthy, but—of course—this is a gross exaggeration of what the study showed. The actual experiment was far more complicated, using a special piece of bike-like equipment that requires fast, intense, 100 percent effort (athletes in their prime can get the weighted fly-wheel moving in two seconds, so the researchers doubled the time for mere mortals) and it wasn't just one four-second burst, it was five four-second bursts with 45 seconds of rest in between and these were repeated every hour. The benefits derived were somewhat lower blood triglycerides and some improvement in fat-burning over the next several hours.

It's an interesting experiment that shows that any movement is better than none at all, but if you're under the impression that a four-second burst of activity—no matter how intense—will give you a healthy body or help you to lose much weight, think again…that's just a pipe dream. This is an ultra-mini-HIIT workout on steroids, so to speak, so if you can get your hands on this special high-resistance bike and use it with faithful dedication, it can be one more little Mini-Workout to add to your weekly total, but you must be aware that it won't replace taking a walk or going for a real bike ride for 20–60 minutes.

Face Aerobics

Whether called Face Yoga, Facerobics, or Facial Toning, facial workouts have had a resurgence of popularity in recent years, but they are nothing new. Jack LaLanne (*the* fitness guru of his time) promoted them in the 1960s and the "lion face pose" has been part of standard yoga practice for eons. How well your face ages is mostly due to genetic luck, eating a healthy diet, drinking plenty of water, and protecting yourself from the sun, but, like all muscles, the 43 muscles in your face can be firm or not-so-firm. While exercising them won't give you more energy or help you live longer, there's evidence that regular "facial workouts" can very modestly reduce the appearance of wrinkles, keep neck and chin slightly firmer, and plump up sagging cheeks a little.

In one of the few controlled studies on face workouts, a group of 40-to-60-year-old women did half-hour face routines every other day for several months. Many of the original participants dropped out (mainly due to boredom, I suspect), but some of those who stuck with it appeared about three years younger after the trial period—so if you're 57 you're going to look maybe 54-ish, not 40 or 45.

Part of me thinks this is just another aggravating way our modern Western culture has found to make us (especially women) feel inadequate so we'll feel pressured to do yet another workout, add yet one more chore to our already overly busy lives, and spend a wad of dough since the "best" results come from high-end spas (according to their ads). However, I recognize that the urge to look attractive is strong, especially in our youth-obsessed culture, so if you have the interest and time, have at it.

I personally would never devote that kind of time to fighting gravity, as the very thought of adding two and a half hours a week to my already full schedule makes me cringe (and furrow my brow!) and I know I'd be absolutely bored to tears spending thirty minutes sitting around making faces—and, believe me, if you have to choose between taking a walk and doing a half-hour face workout, I guarantee the walk will make you look and feel better—but I've seen some mild improvement in my neck from doing the jaw lift fairly often (described below). My BS radar went off when I first heard about it, but I decided to give it a try, since my neck is starting to remind me of my grandmother's (I loved her dearly but would prefer not to emulate her in that particular area). I do a few when showering, as an add-on when doing squat/sit/stands, or at odd moments when I'm positive there's no one around, because they make you look ridiculous…these are the kinds of crazy faces kids love to make and which they find hilarious. However, whether I actually look any better or not, I'll probably keep doing these moves, at least occasionally, as they feel pretty good, help work the kinks out of my neck, and can provide a temporary respite from tinnitus by changing the pressure in the ears.

Here are a few face exercises you can add to a Mini-Workout; if you want to find out more, hit the internet.

- Jaw Lift—bring lower teeth forward and up to touch upper lip, then tip your chin up; hold; relax; repeat; same thing up to corners

- Lion Yawn—open your mouth wide and stick your tongue out and down

- Tongue to Nose—try to touch your nose with your tongue (most won't get much further than the upper lip, but about 10% can make contact; it's called the Gorlin Sign)

- The Trumpet Player—puff out your cheeks one at a time, then both together

- Ear Wiggle—keeping mouth relaxed, wiggle your ears without touching them (or try to)

Please note that you should avoid moves that cause any part of your face to wrinkle...after all, what's the point of smoothing one part if you're deepening the lines on another?

Naturally, your face is exercised constantly in the course of ordinary life, especially if you're an expressive/talkative/emotional person. Jaw and neck muscles can be strengthened simply by chewing gum and giving yourself a daily facial massage while rubbing in moisturizer or sunscreen can do absolute wonders for your complexion. However, if you love to try things and have lots of free time and deep pockets, there are facial exercise "gyms" where someone will massage and stretch and move your face for you; the sessions cost about the same as a massage.

Some degree of vanity is normal, so don't feel guilty about wanting to look your best—although if it's your primary concern in life, you may want to rethink your priorities—but in the long run, in order to feel well, feel good about ourselves, and be happy with who we are, we'd probably all be better off concerning ourselves more with the content of our characters, improving our health, taking care of our families, spending time with friends, being involved in community life, and doing meaningful work, rather than fighting the effects of aging. If you really want to put a smile on your face because you feel happier and more self-assured, go for a walk with a friend and, as William Shakespeare said, "With mirth and laughter, let old wrinkles come."

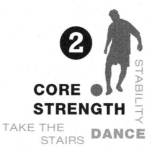

CORE STRENGTH

TAKE THE STAIRS   STABILITY   **DANCE**

Many people think of their core muscles only in terms of having "six-pack abs," and while I'm not immune to the charm of a well-toned tummy (Serena Williams in a crop-top, Emma Stone accusing Ryan Gosling of being photo-shopped in *Crazy, Stupid Love*, Aiden Turner swinging a scythe in *Poldark*, Adam Beach in *Squanto*, Denzel Washington in *The Mighty Quinn*, Nikesh Patel in *Indian Summers*, Mia Hamm, Jackie Chan, Gal Gadot, Lucy Lawless, Beyoncé, The Jonas Brothers, every beach volleyball player on the planet…it's a long beautiful list), core muscles are composed of several sets of interacting muscle groups in both the upper and lower torso that run from the lower abdomen up to the top of the chest, around the sides, and from the upper back down into the gluteus maximus (buttocks), the largest pair of muscles in the human body.

These core muscles perform critical functions, including holding your body upright and keeping your spine healthy and in the proper position. Core muscles enable you to stand, walk, run, ride a bike, jump, or dance. They provide stability when you lift any weight whether it's a barbell or shopping bag, and are what allow you to push or pull something, be it grocery cart, heavy door, stubborn mule, or baby carriage. These are the muscles that let you twist and turn, lift your legs, sit up, roll over in bed, or bend down and pick something up off the floor, from stray feather to case of wine. Your core muscles work just about any time you move at all, and having a strong core is the number one best way to prevent lower back pain and avoid injury. They are critically important muscles and yet many of us do next to nothing to build them up.

The following are some simple exercises and activities to strengthen your core, and the stronger your core, the less likely it is that you'll be plagued with back pain. If you want to do more advanced work (like using weight-machines), team up with a professional trainer for at least a few sessions.

Core strengthening exercises include:

- Toe touches straight up and down and opposite hand to opposite foot with feet shoulder width apart

- Squat/sit/stands

- Bouncing a ball straight up and down and hand to hand

- Walking in water (especially against a current)

- Karate kicks

- Kicking a ball (soccer, kickball)

- Butt squeezes, pelvic tilts, and bridge lifts

- Using stretch bands and weightlifting

- Canoeing, kayaking, rafting, sculling, surfing, paddle-boarding

- Abdominal crunches (these need proper form so you don't hurt your back)

- Seated crunches (reach down to touch the floor, then sit up)

- Using a rowing machine or NordicTrack®

- Hula dancing or hula hooping

- Playing around on a seesaw or swing

- Bike riding either outside or on a stationary bike
- Chopping and carrying wood
- Swiveling your office chair from side-to-side
- Stair climbing and step aerobics
- Taking a deep breath and holding it in for a moment
- Rolling around on a fitness ball
- Baseball and racket sports
- Push-ups, on the floor or against a wall
- Leg lifts and marching in place
- Skateboarding, roller skating, ice-skating
- Jumping on a trampoline
- Dancing (especially something like the twist)
- Gym/health club classes: Pilates, kettlebell, spinning, yoga, Zumba, water aerobics, Pi-Yo
- Any aerobic exercise (works the core as well as heart and lungs)

Any movement where you tighten your mid-section for stability strengthens your core, so any exercise routine can be enhanced by concentrating on tightening abdominals as you move…and here's the perfect place to plug my personal favorite exercise environment, namely any body of water. You can get a fantastic workout without placing stress on joints, so it's ideal for people with arthritis, anyone carrying a lot of extra weight, pregnant women, or those who want more workout time but who are already stressing their joints to the max with other exercise.

Many professional athletes and celebrities use hydro-exercise as an integral part of their workout programs, so they can stay fit without overworking their knees and hips. Natalie Coughlin sprints in the pool, Korey Harris has a YouTube video showing his typical pool routine, and Kareem Abdul-Jabbar runs aqua boot camps; Jennifer Aniston, Christina Milian, Daniel Dae Kim, Nicole Kidman, Natalie Portman, Penelope Cruz, Kerry Washington, and Julia Roberts are all pool devotees. Anyone who thinks exercising or jumping around in a pool is only for wimps hasn't tried it. Swimming and water aerobics engage every muscle in the body for a great workout, and you can't beat canoeing, kayaking, surfing, or paddle boarding for strengthening every pair of core muscles, front and back. Frankly, you get a pretty good core workout even if you're just playing around in the pool, sitting on the edge swinging your legs, or standing at the edge of the ocean keeping your balance as the waves roll in.

If you hate to be cold and only have access to a cold pool, lake, or ocean, get a long sleeve lycra-nylon or neoprene shirt and some tights (they help keep you warm and, not incidentally, are very flattering). Check online for rash-guard clothes, snorkeling gear, swimwear specifically made to hold up in chlorinated water, and/or go to any clothing or sporting goods store and pick up exercise tights and tops made of nylon, spandex, neoprene, or polyester (cotton is slow to dry and doesn't hold up in chlorine).

Please note that if you love the water and make it your regular go-to exercise venue, you still need to engage in some weight-bearing activities to keep bones and joints strong, though it can be as simple as walking and standing instead of sitting. Gravity's impact in the water is approximately 15 percent of what it is on land, so not zero, but in order to stay strong and healthy, you need to spend adequate time with your feet on the ground.

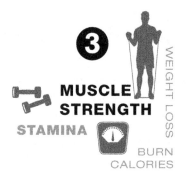

Muscle mass and strength are built by repetitive movements and/or exerting effort against resistance. Well-developed muscles give you stamina, and enable you to perform tasks with ease. Muscles burn more calories than other types of body tissue even at rest, so they really help with weight control. Of course, they look good, too.

You should do simple repetitive movements without any weights every day. I encourage you to do some strength training exercises with hand weights or exercise bands at home at least two times per week, unless you're getting sufficient resistance/weight training exercise at a gym. No specific amount of time for each strength training session is included in these guidelines as it's too idiosyncratic, but you should exert enough effort that by the next day you're aware you've done something, but not enough to be really sore. If you overdo it, your body will let you know quickly, so make note of your weights and reps, and adjust accordingly.

Strength training with weights should not be done more than every other day, no matter how motivated you are to build muscle. This is because lifting weights creates tiny tears in muscle tissue and it is during the "rest and recovery" period that the muscles build up as the little tears repair themselves and grow a bit larger, resulting in increased mass and greater strength. Below is a list of routines and approaches to help you gain strength and avoid injury.

Easy Muscle-Building Moves without Any Added Weight

These can safely be done on a daily basis:

- Any arm and shoulder exercises, especially bicep curls, triceps extensions
- All isometric exercises
- Holding arms straight up or out to the side for an extended period
- All of the movements listed under Seated Exercises for Legs or Butt, Freestanding Leg Exercises, or Full Body Movements

- All walking, but most especially up and down hills or in sand
- Squat/sit/stands are great for building up the largest muscles in the body (glutes and thighs)
- Jogging
- Swimming
- Dancing
- All aerobic exercises
- Canoeing, kayaking, paddleboarding
- Bike riding
- Spinning or stationary bike riding
- Stair climbing
- Repetitive ball bouncing (go hand-to-hand so as to work both arms and side muscles)
- Push-ups (regular, full body, bent knee, or push away from a wall)

Safe Movements with Light Equipment

Depending on your starting point, "light" may be stretchy bands or one-to-five-pound hand weights; it's whatever you can do 10 repetitions of with moderate effort. These can be done two or three times per week:

- Resistance exercise routines using elastic bands can be easily done at home (the bands come with a booklet showing different moves and there are guidelines online; resistance/stiffness varies).

- Working with light hand weights, do any simple arm exercises like bicep curls, overhead reaches, tricep extensions, and side arm presses with a torso twist.

- Add short sets of the same exercises with a higher weight (e.g., if you're using a two-pound weight to do sets of 10 reps, then use a five-pound weight to do a set of 3–5 reps).

- As you get stronger, gradually move up to a slightly higher weight.

Building Muscle Mass with Anaerobic Exercise

This should only be done at a gym with a professional trainer or spotter to help you, and no more often than every other day. Typical routines of lifting very heavy weights as part of a squat-thrust-lift move, in a standing position using arms only, or bench-pressing barbells, will definitely increase strength and the size of muscles, but there is a lot of risk for injury if the movements are done incorrectly. To achieve similar benefits with less chance of hurting yourself, use (what are for you) medium-to-slightly heavy dumbbells/hand weights and "work to failure." This odd expression means you do something like bicep curls until you literally can't do one more; after a rest of a few minutes, you can do another set.

Muscle-Building Movements Using Medium-to-Heavy Equipment

You should work with a trainer until you are experienced with weights. At this level you can do only a few repetitions with a great deal of effort.

- Weightlifting with heavy dumbbells—use these to do a variety of exercises like bicep curls and tricep extensions.

- Lifting barbells—these can be medium or heavy depending on how much weight is added and should only be done with an experienced trainer to assist, guide, and spot you.

- Resistance machines—these are the many different machines found in gyms where you have to exert a lot of effort to move a dead weight (resistance varies depending on how much weight is added); have a trainer show you how to use the equipment properly and help you figure out an appropriate routine.

There are also many weight/resistance machines available for personal use at home. If you decide to go this route, spring for a few sessions with a professional trainer to learn routines and minimize the chance of injury, because if you hurt yourself, the equipment will just become a very expensive clothes rack.

In addition to a wide variety of useful and fun pieces of exercise equipment for sale that can help keep you motivated and safely enhance your workouts, there are also numerous gadgets and pills and potions available in stores and online that are not helpful and/or are downright dangerous, so you must be discriminating. Any product that "absolutely guarantees" that you can soon resemble an Olympic champion without any exercise or change in diet is very obviously something to avoid, but sometimes it's difficult to know if a new piece of training equipment is useful or not. If something sounds absolutely too good to be true (magic pill! magic doo-dad!), avoid it, and if something sounds like it might be a good idea, but you're not sure, do some research. If you can't easily find the information you need, check with the Consumer Product Safety Commission (cpsc.gov) or call up a sports medicine doctor or clinic, as they see the good, the bad, and the ugly every day. Whatever you want to try, please keep in mind this dictum from the Hippocratic Oath: First, do no harm.

Common Activities That Are NOT Recommended

- Wearing ankle and/or wrist weights while exercising (including while walking): although these do add effort to your workout and are very popular, they can put excessive strain on these relatively thin bones and joints, often resulting in injury. If you suffer from osteoporosis or have small bones, you are especially at risk for this kind of mishap. If you want a harder workout, the simplest thing is to pick up your pace, and if you want to add weight(s) while walking, wear a backpack or weighted belt, buy heavier shoes, put stones in your pockets, or get small hand weights you can hold.

- Taking androgens or anabolic steroids: well, they do increase muscle mass, but at a truly terrible cost.

They can cause horrible acne, impotence, man-boobs which are both weird and painful, high blood pressure, baldness, aggression, liver problems, gaps between teeth, depression, and abnormal bone growth. There are many other ways these can ruin your health, but this list should be enough to deter you unless you're an idiot.

In addition to allowing you to better perform daily activities, resistance training improves bone density (or at least slows age-related bone loss), improves coordination, and helps control weight. Given the benefits to be derived from weight training, it's certainly worthwhile to include some in your weekly routine; my recommendation is for a minimum of two to five minutes, twice a week, which is a very modest amount indeed, and if you can do more you will be rewarded.

The biggest problem you're likely to encounter with hand weights if you overdo it is fatigue or muscle soreness, but mistakes with heavy barbells or machines that are not properly adjusted can result in back injuries, pulled muscles, joint problems, and/or sprains, so it's important to work with a pro to learn proper technique. Also, make sure you always warm up before starting any strenuous exercise and take time to stretch afterward.

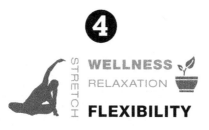

FLEXIBILITY

Other words that come to mind when thinking about flexibility are "supple" and "limber." While we primarily associate these attributes with being graceful and relaxed, these qualities also help prevent injury, improve posture, enhance coordination, minimize joint pain, reduce the risk of injury and lower back problems, and increase circulation—quite a lot of benefit from a little stretching and a few slow deliberate movements.

Stretching is best done when muscles are warm and loose, like they are after exercising; a modest but reasonable goal is three to five minutes of stretching after every walk or exercise class. When your body is relaxed after a warm tub or shower is also a perfect time for some stretching or yoga. Those of us who live with cats or dogs are aware that they always indulge in a good stretch when getting up from one of their frequents naps and often at other times, too, just for the heck of it. If you're stiff after sitting too long and want to emulate your pet by stretching, just loosen up a bit and keep stretches small.

Flexibility is increased by:

- Any routines in the Stretching/Loosening Movements section

- Slow-motion full extension moves—these should be done for every part of the body (e.g., windmill arms making the biggest circles you can)

- Any stretching moves described in the Floor Exercises List

- Yoga moves—if you haven't done yoga before, I recommend a class and/or book or video aimed at the beginner

But...don't do any move to the point of pain—remember, the idea is to stretch and increase your range of motion, not hyperextend a joint and end up incapacitated.

Stretches can be done by:

- Extending a muscle into a good stretch and holding the position for at least 30 seconds (e.g., sitting on the floor with legs straight out in front and reaching as far as possible toward your toes and then holding the position; you will probably be able to feel your muscles relax into the stretch)

- Using your arms or hands to increase a stretch (like bringing one arm across your chest and gently increasing the stretch by pressing with the other arm)

- Stretching against something static (like putting your toe onto a wall and leaning into it)

- Hanging from a jungle gym or monkey bars or dropping your heel off the edge of a step

One last note about stretching: coaches used to recommend intense stretching before any athletic activity or competition (and some still do), but research has shown that not only does this not improve performance, it actually decreases it and can lead to injury. The best way to prepare for intense activity is with low-to-moderate activity that you gradually increase as your muscles warm up.

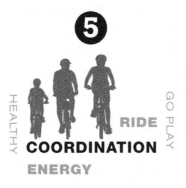

There's a certain level of coordination that's genetic luck, but coordination can always be improved, whether it's hand-eye coordination or how quickly your body is able to respond to mishaps, obstacles, and threats. You may think it doesn't really matter if you're a bit gawky or stiff—and in some regards it doesn't (e.g., it may not affect your job or love prospects)—but in other situations, it matters a great deal: How quickly can you jump out of the way of an out-of-control bicycle? If you bump into something or turn your ankle, will you just stumble, or will you fall? Are you able to recover and catch yourself if you step in a hole? Can your hand zoom up fast enough to protect your face from a flying object? If you look at statistics on injuries, you'll see these are not rare or isolated occurrences and anyone who has spent much time around elderly people knows a fall often results in a broken hip or worse. The good news is that coordination can be improved at any age, and most of the activities that yield the best results are fun—you now have a perfectly valid reason why it's important to take a walk on the beach, shoot some hoops, or just go bounce a ball. The following are some easy activities that enhance coordination and reaction time:

- Playing catch alone or with a partner
- Bouncing a ball from side-to-side
- Kicking a ball and aiming at a target
- Throwing darts

- Playing any sport that requires hitting and catching, like baseball, cricket, or handball

- Shooting hoops

- Playing any racquet sport like tennis, badminton, ping-pong, or racquetball

- Walking on a trail with an uneven surface

- Taking a walk on the beach, especially up and over sand dunes

- Dancing, especially partnered dancing

- Playing Twister and video or Wii™ games that get you up and moving

- Bowling

- Playing volleyball, especially in sand

- Practicing tai chi

- Playing hopscotch

- Juggling

- Hula-hooping

- Surfing or paddleboarding

- Skateboarding

- Playing Frisbee

- Riding a bike in figure eights

- Playing golf or miniature golf

- Doing the limbo

- Taking ballet or modern dance classes

The best way to improve coordination is to participate in the kinds of activities that kids do naturally. When was the last time you said, "I'm going to go out and play?" Here's your excuse, if you need one: go play because it's good for you.

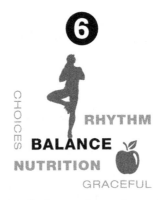

Balance is frequently lumped together with coordination as a single characteristic, and while there is certainly a lot of overlap, they are not exactly the same thing. Many of the activities listed above that help improve coordination will help with balance also—especially racquet sports that require you to shift weight rapidly and where you are frequently in motion with one foot off the ground—but there are a number of movements that focus specifically on balance that can easily be done at home. You don't need to spend a lot of time working on balance alone, but it's worthwhile to dedicate a little time just working on improving your balance during the course of a week.

All balance work engages your core as you make little adjustments to remain steady, but remember, you can always lightly rest a hand on a counter, chair, or wall until you become more secure. Start out with small moves, slowly increasing as you become stronger and more confident. All of the following movements will help improve balance:

- Play around on a giant exercise ball, aka stability ball (follow the instructions that come with the ball, take a class, or do an internet search for ideas)

- When you're changing clothes and doing something like lifting your foot to put your pants on, make your moves slo-mo

- Do tai chi

- Practice ballet moves, working up to an arabesque (leg straight behind with pointed toe, opposite arm lifted in front; at gyms they sometimes call this move an "airplane" because ballet terminology isn't macho enough...um, have you *seen* Mikhail

Baryshnikov?) and when you're comfortable, from this position lean forward until you touch the floor (lightly rest one hand on something or have someone spot you, and if you start to lose your balance, just bend at the knee and put both hands on the floor)

- On hands and knees, lift one leg straight behind you and when steady, lift the opposite arm

- Imitate a flamingo: with palms touching above your head, stand with one knee out to the side and foot lightly pressed against the opposite leg (don't push against the knee)

- Stand on one foot and slowly raise the other leg straight to the side with a flexed foot, then with pointed toe

- As above, but move your leg to the front

- Hook one foot behind the other (you can do this waiting in line anywhere without causing a scene) and just stand around on one leg

- Lift your knee up in front until it's at a 90-degree angle to your hip, hold your arms to the side and when you feel ready, slowly raise your arms higher

- With knees touching, bend one knee and raise your foot straight up in back until leg makes a 90-degree angle; as you become more confident, lift knee up to the side (yes, just like a male dog pee position)

  In the pool:

- Do arm exercises and various swimming strokes while standing on one leg

- With feet shoulder width apart, punch front, side, and across your body with a torso twist using one arm only

- Walk or run first one way and then the other to create a current you can work against

- Make the move you'd use to propel a skateboard, while standing on one leg with knee slightly bent

- With arms out to the side, walk in slow-motion putting one foot directly in front of the other like walking a tightrope

Ta-Da!!! Instant Miraculous Makeover

Once you're in the habit of doing some balance work a few minutes here and there on a regular basis, it will become progressively easier to hold a pose and your body will begin to move a little more gracefully. These improvements will be noticeable but gradual, and you'll be impatient for faster progress. I know you'll be impatient, because that is human nature and it's part of the American psyche to want things to happen quickly. In most areas (e.g., increased muscle strength, improved heart and lung function), there's no way to shortcut the process, but when it comes to balance and looking more attractive, there is something simple you can do that has an immediate transformative effect. Drum roll please...the MIRACLE you've been waiting for! Instantly look and feel better without losing weight or exercising! No pills! No dieting! No restrictions!

What is this marvelous revelation? Sit up straight! Stand up straighter! Yes, just like your mother probably told you a thousand times. Good posture makes you look more attractive and it will absolutely make you feel better too, because a stooping, drooping posture puts a strain on your neck and shoulders and throws your spine out of alignment, often resulting in chronic pain.

Standing with your back straight, chin tilted up, and shoulders back projects an image of self-confidence that others—and you yourself—react to in a positive way. If you want to verify the truth of this, go to any public place, watch people to see how they carry themselves, and observe how other people react to them. Standing up straight makes you appear self-assured, and people who seem poised and confident are considered more attractive by others (and are probably less likely to be bullied). There are numerous studies showing that self-confidence (not conceit, which is quite different) brings success in many areas of life, because what you project to the world and believe about yourself becomes a self-fulfilling prophecy. There's a song by Rodgers and Hammerstein from the 1951 musical *The King and I* that encapsulates this concept perfectly—the idea being that if you pretend to be happy by "whistling a happy tune" in order to fool the people you're afraid of, you'll fool yourself, too—and will soon *be* the self-assured person you are masquerading as. My parents loved musicals and I knew this song well, so as a shy child, I would sing it to myself in order to cope with the fear and uncertainty of new situations. It worked then and it still works now. I'm not shy the way I was as a kid, but I'm still not a natural performer, so when I have to speak in public, I stand up straight, hum a little to myself, and pretend I like it—until I find I do—because I like to talk about the things I feel passionate about.

You probably know that if you force the muscles of your face into a smile—even if you're feeling blue—after a few moments the very act of smiling changes your mood for the better. The smile, in and of itself, starts a chain reaction within you that helps you find humor in a situation or, at the very least, raises your spirit. Good posture is like that too. Holding your head high, standing up straight with shoulders back, and striding purposefully helps you feel better about yourself and helps you find your inner strength. There is a wonderful French phrase, *bien dans sa peau*, that refers to someone who is so comfortable in their own skin that they radiate self-confidence and thus are beautiful to others, even if they don't fit the standard ideal of beauty. If you can pretend to be *bien dans sa peau*, before long, it will be a true reflection of your inner confidence.

Regardless of what other people say, the story you tell yourself about yourself is the most important one you'll ever hear, so…*PSSST*…be careful what you whisper in your own ear…because you're listening.

> *Loving yourself does not mean being self-absorbed or narcissistic, or disregarding others; rather it means welcoming yourself as the most honored guest in your own heart: a guest worthy of respect, a loveable companion.*
>
> —Margo Anand
> French author, teacher,
> writer, and seminar leader

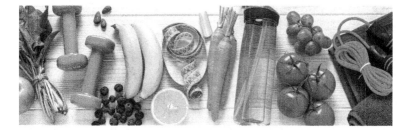

CHAPTER 8

Let's Talk about the Battle of the Bulge

Although the focus of this book is how to incorporate frequent enough movement into daily routines to keep your body functioning well, I recognize that for many people, the motivation to finally get off the couch is being fed up with being overweight. The term "healthy" may be a somewhat vague and squishy concept, but there's nothing vague about the health challenges that often come from carrying a lot of excess weight, such as breathing problems that limit activities, gallbladder disease, joint pain, heart disease, or knees that are giving out. It's also pretty dismaying when you can't wear your own clothes because they no longer fit, and there's no question that in addition to wanting to feel well, it's human nature to want to look good, too. Exercise makes you look and feel more attractive by increasing muscle tone, reducing flab, and flooding your system with happiness hormones. Not incidentally, increased blood flow is tremendously good for your complexion. Every single minute you spend moving helps you look better and improves your mood, while providing your body with the following health benefits:

- Strengthening the heart and increasing lung capacity

- Keeping bones strong

- Lubricating joints (thus reducing pain)

- Helping you feel more confident and in control

- Giving you more energy and stamina

- Helping you sleep better (so you wake up feeling more rested)

- Improving coordination and decreasing the likelihood of a fall

- Lowering blood pressure

- Reducing or preventing acne

- Minimizing wrinkles and flaccid skin

- Helping fight cancers and dementia

- Reducing the risk of developing diabetes

- Boosting the immune system

- Improving mood and sense of well-being

- Minimizing back pain

- Increasing strength and stamina (making everyday chores easier)

If you're worried about the number you see on the scale, regular exercise can help you take off some weight, but remember, muscle weighs more than fat, so it's quite possible that you can be noticeably slimmer and your clothes can be looser, even if your weight doesn't change much. Assuming your diet remains the same as always and you start a moderate exercise program, you will definitely improve muscle tone and yes, you absolutely will lose some weight. Some.

But—and this is a big but—if you want to significantly reduce body fat and be a really healthy version of yourself, you need to make it a regular habit to eat foods that are nourishing and, maybe even more importantly, stop consuming foods that are hardly better than poison, except that instead of killing you quickly, they slowly wreck your health until you just feel like a mess (Public Enemy #1: soft drinks, both regular and diet). And if you literally feel panicky at the thought of giving up junk food treats, it's not because you're weak, it's because they are as addictive as cigarettes and the very act of eating or drinking them sets off a cycle of craving that's very hard to break.

Here in the US (and where we lead, much of the world follows, both for good and ill), we live in a culture where really fattening food is constantly thrust in our faces, where processed-food producers don't have to prove that what they package and promote is good for you, only that it won't kill you outright, and where 24/7 we are exposed to advertisements encouraging us to consume food and drink that is just terrible for our health. Advertisers are brilliant at pushing the buttons that drive our desires so that we'll spend our dollars buying their products again and again.

And let's face it, a lot of junk food is very tasty. Once we've gotten in the habit of eating it, the unconscious parts of our brains that signal pleasure and desire light up at the very sight of it. A great deal of research goes into finding the magic combinations of sugar, salt, fat, preservatives, dyes, artificial ingredients, lab-created "natural" flavors, and just the right blend of textures, so we will continuously eat w-a-a-a-a-y more than we need and still want more, more, more.

The inescapable conclusion is that if you really want to feel well and be well, you have to mostly eat food that's good for you...and I'm guessing you already have a pretty good idea of what that looks like: a variety of fresh fruits and vegetables, nuts, seeds, legumes, whole grain products, foods that are high in fiber, herbs and spices, seafood, eggs, lean-ish meat (and not too much), and of course, you need to drink plenty of water.

Although there's plenty of debate about what constitutes the very healthiest approach to eating (pescatarian, Mediterranean diet, vegetarian, vegan, flexitarian, low fat, Blue Zones diet, no dairy, olive oil versus canola versus coconut oil, DASH, low carbohydrate, Paleo, gluten free, Okinawan diet, etc.), there is not a single responsible parent or medical source in the entire world that says in order to be healthy you should eat trans fats, high fructose corn syrup and artificial sweeteners, or lard-laden, extremely salty, chemically enhanced, highly processed, super sweet, fiber-free foods that give you two, three, or four times your recommended daily calorie intake.

In order to achieve and maintain good health, you need to make sure you eat nutritious foods (at least the majority of the time), drink sufficient water every day, get enough sleep, and keep sugary treats and junk food to a level where they don't overwhelm your system. Being plumper than a fashion model doesn't mean you're overweight, but if you're carrying enough extra pounds that you don't feel well or it's hard to accomplish certain normal activities (like bending over to tie your shoes), you need to be careful not to get to the point where you are seriously endangering your health. And, of course, you need to get plenty of exercise on a regular basis, because unfortunately it's not optional: if you're not pumping oxygen-rich blood to all the parts of your body, it cannot perform its many different jobs properly, and you cannot be healthy.

If nutritious foods rarely appear on your plate and the majority of your calories come from fatty meats and fried food, or candy, sodas, sugary cocktails, and other super-sweet junk, the outlook for a reasonably healthy old age is poor indeed. That kind of diet can clog arteries, overwhelm the liver, feed cancer cells, raise blood pressure, cause tooth decay and bad skin, and sooner or later may lead to diabetes, heart problems, gout, and/or a stroke.

The irresistible drive to overeat is only partly due to the fact that junk foods taste good and look appealing. A ton of research into various food additives (high-fructose corn syrup and artificial sweeteners in particular) has shown that many of the additives themselves are addictive and drive subconscious cravings in the same ways that addictive drugs do. So yes, sure, it's your hand that's reaching for the junk food instead of the apple, but it's not entirely your fault. It's not easy to wean yourself off of junk food, but it is definitely possible...and definitely worth the effort.

WHAT HAPPENS TO ALL THE CALORIES YOU EAT?

The recommended daily number of calories is 2,000 for the average adult woman, and 2,500 for the average adult man. How do those calories get used up each day?

Let's see what happens to a hypothetical man—we'll call him Joe—who consumes exactly 2,500 calories every day, which totals 17,500 per week. Joe is not a professional athlete, but he exercises on a regular basis.

Calories that Joe burns weekly by exercising:

1,500	Running five miles three days per week
200	Lifting weights two days a week
2,100	Walking his dog Sparky every morning and every evening
200	Riding a stationary bike in front of the TV twice a week
4,000	TOTAL

Wow! Joe is a super-disciplined guy and is burning up 4,000 calories every week by exercising...but what happens to the other 13,500?

Approximately 800 calories are required each day to maintain Joe's body temperature at a steady 98.6 degrees and another 400 or so are needed to keep his brain working. Some calories are burned by the behind-the-scenes activities of breathing, digesting food, pumping blood, etc., but the majority are burned up fueling the activities of daily life: working, cooking, fidgeting, walking around, playing with Sparky, making the bed, shopping, standing up, doing laundry, washing the car, cleaning the house, etc.

So yes, exercising burns calories and is really helpful for increasing strength and stamina (and health in general), but most of the calories used each day go toward fueling normal activities (what researchers refer to as "Non-Exercise Activity Thermogenesis," aka NEAT). So it's easier to reach or maintain a healthy weight—even if you don't consistently exercise as rigorously as Joe (and very few of us do)—if you keep steadily on the go much of the day and bump up the level of doing ordinary things with Mini-Workouts throughout the day, every day.

INSPIRATION IS ALL AROUND, BUT MOTIVATION IS WITHIN

Even if the desire to lose weight is really your primary motivation for wanting to get into better shape, you may not be mentally ready to revamp your diet right now, even if you are well aware of the fact that there's a lot of room for improvement. As you incorporate Mini-Workouts into your schedule and embark on a walking program, remember that your goal is to be happier and healthier for the long term, not to exhaust yourself or drive yourself nuts trying to make too many changes all at once. However, if you'd like to lose some weight—even if you're postponing a diet overhaul until some future date—there are some fairly painless modifications you can probably make that will improve your health and help you shed some weight fairly easily, if you know where to look. Analyze your typical weekly fare and see if there are one or two habits you could shift; with a little creativity, you can often find a less caloric substitute for something you enjoy on a regular basis, without much, if any, sacrifice. Check out the many resources online or at the bookstore or library for ideas about recipe substitutions that will scratch some flavor or texture itch but with fewer calories or a better nutrition profile.

A lot of people consume a huge proportion of their weekly calorie intake in liquid form; however, liquids don't fill you up the way solid foods do, so if you're in the habit of consuming high-calorie drinks, you could potentially save thousands of calories every week just by changing what's in your glass. Sodas, both regular and diet, have been repeatedly shown to be detrimental for both weight and health, so a simple switch to iced tea, lemonade, chocolate almond milk, or club soda with a splash of fruit juice could potentially improve your health very quickly, and finding other lower calorie substitutions may be easier than you think. For example, if you go out every Friday night with a group of friends for TGIF margaritas, you could easily save a ton of calories just by switching to a less fattening drink while you relax with friends and celebrate the end of the workweek. Since bar and restaurant margaritas range from around 300 up to 850 per drink, two or three can add up to half or more of the total number of recommended calories for an entire day. If you were to have an equivalent quantity of Scotch or vodka and soda instead (especially if it's heavy on the soda), a Bloody Mary on the rocks, or a beer or glass of wine (or lite beer or a wine spritzer for even more savings), you'll be much better off. If you're a milk drinker, if you were to switch from whole milk at 150 calories per cup to a plant-based milk at around 30 calories per cup, at one cup every day, you'd have an instant savings of 840 calories per week, and barely notice (once you get used to a new milk, you might even find you like it better...I did, much to my surprise).

If you usually drink a large glass of orange juice every morning, try replacing the juice with a whole orange a few days a week (Cara-cara navels are my favorite) and see if there's an orange-flavored tea you like that you can drink with your meal instead of straight OJ, or try a combination of half tea and half orange juice…you can think of it as the breakfast version of an Arnold Palmer. If you typically go to a coffee bar every afternoon for a Mo-cha-Frappa-Macchiato-Caramel treat, you may easily be consuming 1,500–4,000 calories each week just so you can get out of the office for a few minutes and/or so you can get an afternoon caffeine boost. If you bring a Shake-Up from home instead (the recipe below is from my book on healthy eating), you can still enjoy a creamy milkshake-like treat that probably has less than a 10th of the calories (not to mention 10 times the nutrition) and you can still go out for a walk and grab a coffee if your goal is really a mental break and change of scene. You may be skeptical, but if you try it, I think you'll be very happy you did.

LUISA'S (MILK) SHAKE-UPS

Creamy, cold, sweet, flavorful, and perfect for sucking through a straw, milkshakes are delicious and fun. Alas, made the usual way with ice cream and syrup, they are strictly off-limits for anyone trying to limit calories. The majority of fast food shakes are even worse—they are bad not only for your waistline, but for your entire body. A few years ago, *The Guardian* newspaper ran a funny but scary piece with the headline "The 59 Ingredients in a Fast Food Strawberry Milkshake," which listed all 59 of them (disodium phosphate, methylphenyl-glycidate, methyl benzoate, and 56 other unpronounceable chemicals). However, two ingredients were notably absent: strawberries and milk. While not all fast food shakes are equally terrible, they are all to be diligently avoided, both for the unknown chemicals they may contain and for the outrageously high calorie counts that range from 600 up to 1,680 (!), with the average being around 1,200 per serving.

The recipe on page 149 meets all the requirements for taste and sensory pleasure while delivering lots of nutrition and almost no sugar or fat. Incidentally, this shake will last a couple of days in the fridge and still be creamy. It thickens as it stands, so if it gets too thick, add some ice or milk and give it another whirl in the blender. All milkshakes should be served really cold, in an appropriately tall, cheerful glass. Once good and cold, Shake-Ups can be put into an insulated container and taken on the road; just give it another shake before drinking.

RECIPE for Chocolate Shake-Up

6-8 servings

1 cup vanilla yogurt

2 cups (1 lb block) silken tofu

1 cup unsweetened vanilla non-dairy milk

1 large banana (or chunks of frozen banana)

1 TB unsweetened cocoa powder

2 tsp vanilla

1 TB roasted beets (leftovers or from the salad bar at the grocery store)

   (Do *not* use pickled beets)

2 TB rinsed white beans, aka cannellini (may substitute black or red beans)

1 (4 oz) jar prune puree or baby food (or 4-6 dried plums, aka prunes)

2-3 packets of stevia (or equivalent sweetener)

DIRECTIONS

Put all ingredients into a blender pitcher and blend on high speed until frothy. Chill well. If serving immediately, add a few ice cubes to the mix to get it cold enough.

Optional: Top with a sprinkling of cinnamon, nutmeg, date sugar, or a light grating of dark chocolate.

Make it vanilla: Leave out the cocoa, beets, and prunes and add an extra teaspoon of vanilla extract.

The version above is the most nutritious (also my favorite), but this recipe is very stable and forgiving, so quantities do not need to be exact and you can easily adjust it to suit your taste. Or if you're out of something, you can still make it and it will be fine. Don't like banana? No problem, leave it out. No white beans in the house? Ditto. No vanilla yogurt? No biggie, just add some plain yogurt and up the vanilla extract. One last word on the ingredients: the concept of adding roasted beets may seem whacko, but if you remember that most processed sugar comes from sugar beets, it doesn't seem so odd; they add a sweetness and depth of flavor that's really good and the shake doesn't even vaguely taste like beets (I got the idea from my friend, teacher and cookbook author Marlene Sorosky Gray, who uses them in the best chocolate cake I ever had). Enjoy!

This recipe is just one example of how you can swap one treat for another without suffering if you put your creative thinking cap on. You may find that, on balance, you like the new version even better since it allows you to have a special treat every day and not feel the least bit guilty about it. Focus on making choices that feed your body what it needs to thrive every day.

I had to grow to love my body.

I did not have a good self-image…
finally it occurred to me,

I'm either going to love me or hate me.

And I chose to love myself. Then
everything sprung from there.

Things that I thought weren't
attractive became sexy.

Confidence makes you sexy.

—Queen Latifah

American rapper, singer,
songwriter, actress,
and producer

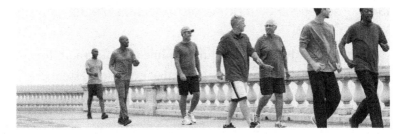

CHAPTER 9

Scheduling Walking and Aerobic Exercise

The human body is designed for bipedal locomotion, so in order to be reasonably healthy, you should aim to walk at least two and a half hours a week on a regular basis. The US Department of Health and Human Services recommends a minimum of 150 minutes/week of aerobic exercise (like brisk walking or any other similar level activity) OR 75 minutes/week of vigorous exercise (running/jogging/aerobic dancing) AND two (short) sessions per week of some kind of strength training; further along are some suggestions for easily adapting your schedule to make room for these activities. You already know that exercise is essential for maintaining a healthy heart, for revving up the metabolism to burn stored fat, and for adding more muscle (so you not only get stronger, but burn more calories even at rest), but exercise also provides hidden benefits that you may not be aware of.

- Strengthening bones—all weight-bearing activities help keep bones strong, thus reducing the risk of breaking one due to a fall or other accident, and helps minimize the likelihood of getting osteoporosis

- Reducing stress and boosting mood and self-esteem—"feel good" chemicals called endorphins are released during exercise; this is sometimes referred to as a "runner's high," but you don't have to run to get it

- Improving sleep—experts have found that people who exercise, no matter what time of day, sleep better than those who don't (they used to tell you not to exercise too close to bedtime, but for most people it's not an issue, so go ahead and ride your exercise bike in front of the TV if evening is the best time for you)

- Improving memory and brain function—neural connections develop during exercise, keeping reasoning skills sharp, and researchers believe that people who exercise have a lower risk of developing Alzheimer's disease and other types of dementia than those who don't

- Reducing illness—increased oxygen strengthens the immune system, helping you to ward off viruses and infections

- Lowering the risk of diabetes and some cancers—your body becomes more efficient at regulating insulin and clearing sugar from the blood (and sugar feeds some cancer cells)

- Minimizing aches, pains, and stiffness—moderate exercise strengthens and aligns the whole musculoskeletal system, and there's nothing like stretching and/or yoga to work out kinks and keep you limber

- Improving the digestive system—moving is essential for keeping the gastrointestinal tract working properly, and can even help with liver disease or irritable bowel syndrome

WALKING AS A REGULAR HABIT AND SCHEDULING OTHER EXERCISE

Regular exercise needs to be an integral part of your weekly routine, and once it becomes habit, as with all habits, you won't want anything to get in the way of accomplishing it. Establishing new habits takes some effort and a plan, but if you can push past the three-week mark, your new routine will begin to transform itself into your new habit, eventually turning into one that you will embrace with all the tenacity with which you currently keep your rear end glued to a chair.

Turning Mini-Workouts into habit is surprisingly easy because once you've linked an exercise to an activity, you have frequent reinforcement. You're repeating the same activity in the same place, over and over again (e.g., doing 15 squat/sit/stands every time you go to the bathroom, since you go to the bathroom numerous times a day). Mini-Workouts also easily become ingrained habits because you can see improvements very quickly since you're dealing with such small numbers. For example, maybe at first you can only do 5 squat/sit/stands in a set, but after four days you're able to do 7 at a time; after ten days you're up to 9; within two weeks you can do 12; in three weeks, perhaps 15 at a time and once a day you can push through to 25 repetitions. Maybe you can't imagine doing that number of reps, but you'll soon find you can, and once you can, you'll want to do it again…and believe it or not, you'll be happy about it.

You can see how easy it is to turn Mini-Workouts into a regular habit. But having your two and a half hours a week of walking or other aerobic exercise become so ingrained that it becomes second nature may be a bit trickier both because you don't have the sheer number of reinforcements, and because the numbers are a little squishier (did you walk 27 or 34 minutes? Did you maintain a steady pace or were there distractions that slowed you down?), so you must create a schedule that is consistently doable week in and week out. The schedule can be any combo that works for you—and then you really, really, really have to stick to it. Don't decide day by day if you'll walk at lunchtime or wait until after work…by which time you're tired and may decide "not today," and then the next day you're "not in the mood," and the next thing you know, you've abandoned it altogether.

Any one of the following schedules will get you to two and a half hours a week, so just pick one.

- Five days a week you take a 30-minute walk in the morning (if necessary, get up earlier or ditch some other activity to make time)

- Five days a week take a 15-minute walk in the morning and a 15-minute walk in the evening

- Five days a week you take a 10-minute walk in the morning, a 10-minute walk midday, and a 10-minute walk in the evening (if you're only going for 10 minutes, try to set a good pace right from the start)

- Six days a week you walk five times a day for five minutes (this is a schedule for people who can't do more at one go for health reasons; ideally, you'll be working your way up to a minimum of 10 minutes per walk)

- Three days a week take a 15-minute walk in the morning, a 15-minute walk in the evening, and then go for a one-hour hike sometime on the weekend

- One day a week do an hour of a scheduled class (aerobics, water aerobics, dance, spinning) plus three days a week you take a 30-minute walk

- Once a week you play basketball, soccer, or tennis for an hour (and really keep moving the whole time) and three days a week you walk for 30 minutes

- Twice a week take a 45-minute aerobic-level class, plus twice a week go for a 30-minute walk

- Two or three times a week ride your bike to work or school and then schedule walks to bring the total up to two and a half hours

- Twice a week take a one-hour class, and once a week go for a 30-minute walk

Though playing sports or being a gym-rat are absolutely not requirements for good health, if you can find a structured activity you enjoy and that gets you moving it will be helpful, as there's no question that most of us work harder in a class environment than when left to our own devices. If you haven't exercised in a long time and don't even know what to try, think about what you liked as a kid. For example, if you enjoyed biking, ride a bicycle or try a beginners' spinning class; if you loved canoeing at camp, find a rowing group to join or buy a rowing machine and put it in front of the television.

If there is a convenient and affordable health club, YMCA, or gym nearby, great; if not, virtually every community has some kind of recreation department or classes that are offered through the community college or senior center. Use social media, Craigslist, or check out bulletin boards at libraries and universities, etc., to find like-minded folks if your friends and family have different interests or, worse, discourage you from exercising. The reality is that fitness levels and diet habits are frequently very similar within family and friend groups and if you make the decision to start exercising or cut out junk food, you may encounter a fair amount of unconscious resistance from those who are close to you. If someone wants you to engage in a sedentary activity when you want to go for a walk, have a comment ready that's hard to refute, explaining that you're trying to get your cholesterol or blood pressure down to a certain number. If you express a concrete concern about a specific health issue, the people who care about you are less likely to try and talk you out of your new exercise regimen.

Whatever you choose, make sure it's convenient, even if it means spending a little extra money. If it's a pain to get to a club or class, your enthusiasm will wane and you'll find reasons not to go (bad weather, too tired, it's too far, don't feel like fighting traffic, can't get a cab, unreliable bus route, etc.). I'm sympathetic if cost is a limiting factor, but find creative ways to get around it, like working part-time at a health club in exchange for membership (also a great way to start hanging out with people who care about fitness) or buying a secondhand health club lifetime membership on a resale site. If you're free during the middle of the day, some clubs offer off-peak special rates or lower rates for seniors. And when you're doing the financial calculation, remember that healthy people spend much less money than sickly people on doctors and medications and miss work far less often, which is why many insurance programs and businesses offer to pay all or some of the fees for health club membership (check with your H.R. department if you have one). If you're part of an HMO, they may offer free or low-cost classes since they know that people who actively pursue wellness are less likely to need healthcare.

If you're afraid you can't keep up in a dance-type class, take a spin class or do water aerobics so you can go at your own pace; you won't slow down the rest of the class, and if you're really a klutz, it doesn't matter because no one can see you under water. Mortified at the idea of being in public in a bathing suit? Get some lycra-nylon tights, shirt, or jacket to put over your suit (very flattering, plus they really help keep you warm) and you can always get a robe or big towel to wear to the edge of the pool for modesty.

One more thing: You may not want to exercise around other people because you think they will judge you or look down on you because you're overweight or out of shape, but the truth is that when someone new joins a class, no matter their shape, most people think, "good for you," and, besides, a year or two earlier, many of the fit people you see may have been where you are now. And if anyone makes a hurtful or insulting comment, just ignore them and recognize that they are rude and insensitive. Your goal is to focus on your own health and well-being and to keep getting progressively stronger, so don't let someone else's arrogant attitude determine what you will or won't do.

If going to a class is not an option or if you absolutely hate gyms, then set up a walking schedule that works and remember, this is not the time for a heel dragging stroll, but an arm-swinging, hip-waggling pace that will raise your heart rate—it can be in a park, on a track or treadmill, or just around the block—and the only thing you really need is a decent pair of shoes and maybe some good headphones. If possible, take some of your walks outside where you can enjoy—and be energized by—the beauty of nature. In Japan, much of the population engages in what's called *shinrin-yoku*, which translates to "forest-bathing." The idea is that when you are surrounded by the beauty of the natural world, you will find peace of mind and respite from the pressures of modern living. Even if you don't have a handy forest, you can probably find a park, beach, botanical garden, golf course, vineyard, community garden, or lakefront trail where you can take your vigorous walk and then do some deep breathing and relaxation at the end while "bathing" in a virtual or actual forest.

Though most cities have numerous parks and gardens, if you're in an area where it's not feasible for you to walk there, plan a route that will end up at a fountain or pocket park and let your eyes rest on something green, even if only for a few minutes. If being outside isn't a good option due to bad weather or some other reason, get a treadmill or stationary bike and set it up in front of a TV (and put a plant in view); if you find it boring, or need extra motivation, make a pact with yourself that you may watch some totally indulgent show that's a secret pleasure, but only while walking.

Find Walking Partners

If you connect with a walking partner you'll walk farther, more often, and will enjoy it more. My best walking buddy is Eileen, and we were brought together because our dogs fell in love at the park. Eileen is younger than I am and her natural pace is faster than mine, so we go at my pace, not hers, but we have fun and keep each other entertained and motivated, our dogs absolutely love it, and we've become really good friends as we walk and talk. My husband John and I enjoy frequent walks together, but when he really wants a challenging aerobic workout since he's tall-ish and I'm short-ish, his walking partner is his friend and co-worker Mary Beth, who is tall and fit, and can match him stride for stride. They often walk to work together (four+ miles each way) and treat themselves to a cappuccino at the end; they get a good workout, strengthen their friend-ship, and can talk about what's going on at the office with-out the usual constraints.

You can undoubtedly find an established walking/ hiking group in your area through social media, but if you don't find one that fits your schedule, you can easily start your own. My friend Sharon wanted a way to meet smart women of a certain age, plus get more exercise, so she asked a few friends if we were interested and we said yes; then we each asked three to four others and bam! Club or-ganized. Each month one person selects a hike, sends out directions and details, and then those who want to come just show up, no RSVP necessary. I've met some interest-ing women and seen some beautiful trails I might not have discovered on my own. One acquaintance has a city walk-ing group that calls themselves the Jabber-Walkers—fairly self-explanatory—and when I meet my friend Gail at the park, she describes what we do as "power-talking" and it's a much healthier get together (not to mention cheaper) than just meeting for lunch. Other friends have found walking partners at Weight Watchers meetings; obviously, everyone is there for the same reason and you can be sure every person there needs to up their walking routine.

Another option for finding an organized walking group is to look for local "Moai Walking Groups," which are social/walking clubs that are an outgrowth of the Blue Zone approach to living a healthy life (*moai* means "meeting for a common purpose" in Japanese). In the November 2005 cover story of National Geographic, writer Dan Buettner looked at five specific regions in the world where the populations live longer than average and where many live to be 100 years old or more. He analyzed the attributes of these disparate cultures—Sardinia, Italy; Okinawa, Japan; Loma Linda, California; the Nicoya Peninsula, Costa Rica; Icaria, Greece—and found that one of the common threads was daily moderate physical activity, even though going to a health club is almost unheard of in these various locales...in other words, the normal mode of transportation is walking from one place to the next, and all of these places are hilly. (The other points in common are little or no smoking, putting family ahead of other concerns, a vegetarian or semi-vegetarian diet, high consumption of legumes—beans like chickpeas/garbanzos, cannellini, black beans, soybeans, lentils, and navy beans—on a regular basis, and being socially active and integrated into the community. "Blue Zone" living has become a movement; for more information: www.bluezones.com).

Since we are strongly influenced by those with whom we spend a lot of time, it will be really helpful if you can find walking and exercising pals, even if it means moving a little bit out of your comfort zone. If you'd like to get a treadmill or alternate your walks with other things like paddling or biking but money is an issue, head to Craigslist, eBay, a neighborhood info/exchange website, or see if there's a sporting goods equipment resale store in your area. I live in Napa Valley, California, where we have several bicycle touring companies that buy all new equipment every year, so at the end of tourist season they sell their entire stock of high-quality bicycles for a fraction of the retail price; many kayak/canoe rental places do the same. When you start to think outside the retail-store box, there are bargains to be found. If you frequently exercise on your own, treat yourself to some of the latest exercising gadgets, good headphones (but keep the volume down and use good judgment if you walk or run where there's traffic), and anything else that will help keep you going, like apps for smartphones, participation in online communities, and playlists of your favorite music. Hit the internet to visit sites like www.everybodywalk.org for maps, tips, advice, and inspiring videos. Take a look at what may be available on your phone for free (I only recently figured out that the step-counter on my phone is much more accurate than the old gadget I have that clips to my belt), or maybe get a fitness tracker to help keep you motivated; they can readily be found secondhand, often still in the box.

OTHER ACTIVITIES THAT GET YOU MOVING

Your schedule undoubtedly includes plenty of chores and errands you have to do each week, but don't feel guilty about scheduling in time to enjoy activities that get you moving, even if they don't seem absolutely essential. Recognize that your own mental and physical health are as important as anyone else's, and keep in mind that if you have a lot of responsibility caring for others, you'll do a better job in the long run if you make it a priority to take care of yourself, too. It's important to be realistic about how much benefit is derived from various activities, so take a look at your weekly schedule and see where you may need to make a few tweaks or adjustments—or what chores you can delegate to someone else so you can thrive (maybe have your groceries delivered so you can take time to go for a swim or play golf).

Playing Sports

Many people think that because they play a sport on the weekend, they don't need to get any exercise during the week. But the truth is that the more intense your "weekend warrior" activities, the more important it is to get other regular exercise during the week in order to prevent injury. Additionally, weekend activities often include beer or pizza afterward, so the net outcome for health can easily be in the negative column. This is not to say give it all up, but to say think it through. If you play sports on the weekend, that's great, but keep in mind that you need to move every day to stay in decent shape so you won't get injured, and make sure your post-game celebratory meal is something nutritious except on very rare occasions.

Beyond whatever playtime you manage on the weekends, there are plenty of ways to work some aerobic exercise into your week, whether it's riding a bike, skateboarding, or playing ping-pong. If these are counted as part of your two and a half hours of aerobic exercise per week, then they absolutely must be scheduled in—for example, every Tuesday you ride your bike to the farmers market, or every Friday, without fail, you play tennis. If these kinds of activities are random and unplanned, then they must be in addition to the two and a half hours of exercise on your weekly agenda.

Shopping, Errands, Chores

You may be a generally busy person and thus think that your many miscellaneous activities can take the place of walking, aerobics classes, or sports, but most can't. A few minutes here and there of moving from Point A to Point B is certainly better than just sitting, but you must be active enough to elevate your heart rate and sustain it for a minimum of 15 minutes to get real aerobic benefit, and 20-to-60-minute sessions are even better. So, unfortunately, unless you're zooming around a warehouse store without stopping, shopping doesn't count, and an activity like washing a car only counts if you're really using sustained vigorous movements for 15 minutes or more. When you're on your feet, you do get the benefits of weight-bearing activity which helps keep bones strong, but walking slowly, standing around, or doing the museum shuffle will not get your heart rate up enough to improve heart and lung function.

Gardening

This is one of the few ordinary household activities that is frequently aerobic—the only people who don't think gardening is hard work are people who don't do it. Gardening can work well as a shared chore if you can find the right partner, especially for something that doesn't require all your attention like weeding or pruning a hedge where you can work side-by-side and chat. If you can't find a buddy, indulge in some good headphones and enjoy being outside. A side note—don't be shy or overly frugal about hiring someone to do a task that can throw your back out, because nothing derails getting in shape like an injury. Personally, while I still enjoy planting a summer vegetable garden, pruning the hedge along the driveway, and the occasional weed-pulling session, I just can't/don't/won't dig big holes or schlep rocks anymore. To borrow a phrase from *Sex and the City*, sometimes you just have to throw money at a problem so you can get on to the parts you like. If you pace yourself, you can work outside for hours, get a great workout, have fun, and create a beautiful or bountiful garden. The added bonus is that it is very rewarding to eat food you have grown yourself, and by definition that means you'll be eating healthy fruits and vegetables since you can't grow your own junk food.

If you live in an apartment and have a balcony, you can plant a vertical garden (hit the web for some very creative design ideas), organize with other tenants to put planter boxes on the roof of your building, or see about joining or volunteering at a community garden.

Remember, whatever Mini-Workouts you link to routines, whatever walking schedule works for you, whatever classes you want to take, whatever sports you like to play, whatever you decide works for you to get going and keep moving, make it doable and fun, because...

> *It's not what we do once in a while that shapes our lives, it's what we do consistently.*
>
> —Tony Robbins
> Author, coach,
> philanthropist,
> and motivational speaker

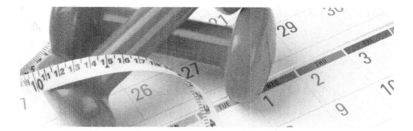

CHAPTER 10

Mapping Your Move-All-Day Schedule

Once you've figured out which Mini-Workout exercises you like and when you like to do them *and* have mapped out a walking plan for yourself that specifies where and when you will walk, it's a good idea to write up a weekly schedule. The simple act of writing down your plan will help your unconscious self make a commitment to keep it. Below are some suggestions for how you might incorporate movement into your daily schedule that will benefit your health and well-being in subtle and not-so-subtle ways.

ON WEEKDAYS

- In bed before getting up—awaken and flex and loosen your body (and do your Kegel exercises).

- Brushing teeth + morning ablutions—your personal Mini-Workout that you can safely do in the bathroom. Start the day with a set of squat/sit/stands.

- Getting dressed—do a few toe touches and arm exercises, work on balance, and do some full range of motion moves.

- At breakfast time—your personal limited-space kitchen Mini-Workout while waiting for microwave/toaster/coffee; later in the morning during coffee or tea breaks, remember to move around.

- Take a morning walk several times a week (or every day…it's a wonderful way to get your body warmed up and your brain in gear).

- After using the toilet—a set of squat/sit/stands and/or your personal limited-space bathroom Mini-Workout.

- The morning commute—small seated limited-space movement exercises (if too embarrassed by something like a bicep curl, just quietly do butt squeezes). No commute? Do some floor exercises.

- Morning at the office or wherever—use a bathroom you have to walk to and do a set of squat/sit/stands every time you go.

- Throughout the day, take random breaks to walk around and roll your shoulders any time you feel stiff; take stairs when you can.

- While at your desk—do some chair exercises and remember to get up often just for the heck of it.

- Walk around when you use the phone; use a stand-up desk or worktable from time to time if that's an option.

- Mid-morning in the office (or home) kitchen getting water, coffee, tea, or when having a (healthy) snack break—your personal limited-space kitchen Mini-Workout.

- On days when you're busy at home doing chores, play can't-sit-still music.

- Lunchtime—your kitchen Mini-Workout + a walk, run errands, and do arm exercises, shoulder rolls + neck/back stretches to keep from getting too stiff.

- Indulge in a midday walk several times a week.

- Your afternoon routines—squat/sit/stands every time you use the lavatory; chair exercises; get up often just to move around; walk down the hall.

- On your commute home—seated small movement exercises.

- After work—go for a walk, walk your dog, and take an exercise class or go out and ride your bike.

- Waiting for hot water for shower or bath—your (safe) bathroom step routine and toe touches, arm reaches, or squat/sit/stands.

- When warmed up from bathing is a great time for yoga or meditation (even if you have to make dinner, you can probably carve out at least five or ten minutes for some "me time").

- Changing into comfy clothes for the evening—flex fingers and toes, work on balance, do some floor exercises, and/or stretching.

- After dinner—do some flexing/loosening movements, and this is a great time to take a stroll if conditions permit.

- Watching TV in the evening—ride an exercise bike or walk on a treadmill; do arm exercises with hand weights.

- Brushing teeth + before bed ablutions—your personal bathroom Mini-Workout plus some stretching.

- Close your eyes, roll your shoulders, and do some deep breathing to quiet your mind for sleep.

ON WEEKENDS

- Any or all of your weekday Mini-Workouts, plus a long walk, bike ride, swim, round of golf, or go canoeing or kayaking.

- If you belong to a gym, get the weekend off to a great start with a Saturday morning class or become part of a hula-hooping or tai-chi in the park group.

- Organize or join an activity like going for a hike or playing a sport—try to do at least one activity that gets you moving outside, and if it's something you can do with friends, so much the better (bocce, doubles tennis, shooting hoops).

- Walk your dog or a neighbor's dog or volunteer to walk the dogs at your local shelter; volunteer with a horse therapy group and/or go riding.

- If you play a sport or go watch your kids play a game, stay on your feet and keep moving rather than just sitting around watching other people do stuff.

- When running errands, instead of driving, walk from one store to the next and/or park further away; use time waiting for a cashier to work on balance.

- If you go to a mall, take stairs to change levels, walk back to your car to deposit packages.

- Play dance music and do your weekend chores with gusto (cleaning the house, folding laundry, working in the garden, or washing the car).

- If you play tennis or go bowling, remember to keep moving while waiting for other people to fetch a ball or take their turn.

- Go dancing! If you have a partner who likes to dance, great; if not, there are line-dancing events, square-dance groups, or clubs where you can just jump in and dance by yourself or with a group of friends.

- When attending a special event (sports, concert, movie), think what you might do, such as seated exercises, work on balance while standing in line, offer to go get snacks, and park some distance from the entrance.

WHEN YOU CHOOSE MOVEMENT, YOU CHOOSE WELL-BEING

Think about how many opportunities there are every day when you can incorporate movements into your schedule: while watching TV (bike, treadmill, weights); the numerous sets of squat/sit/stands you could do by linking a set to your bathroom breaks; the many extra steps that can be added just by walking a bit farther five or 10 times a day; how taking stairs instead of an escalator or elevator can work your glutes; how commute time can be used for butt squeezes, isometric strengthening, and the like; how time spent waiting for something in the kitchen could easily be spent working a body part; and all the many opportunities you have every day to move your body instead of sitting like a lump or standing like a marble statue.

You can see how these random moments here and there can add up to quite a lot of time and a meaningful number of reps…and all these movements will reduce joint pain, help prevent stiffness, improve muscle tone, keep your brain more alert, and increase circulation, which benefits every part of your body from heart and lungs to skin and teeth.

Though you are making a serious commitment to stick to the movement schedule you establish, realistically, there will be days when you are super busy and can't keep to your plan or you slack off just because you're not in the mood. When those days happen and you don't hit 100%, don't berate yourself and give up, just give yourself a pat on the back for what you did manage and, on the days when your lazy self reigns supreme, a little kick in the pants to do more tomorrow. For good or ill, "getting healthy" is not something you take care of once and then check off your to-do list—it's an ongoing process with ups and downs...and ups and downs—so recognize that over the course of time you will likely need to rededicate yourself periodically to the habits that lead to a healthier body and a sense of well-being.

- Do an honest self-assessment. If necessary, forgive yourself.

- Stop wishing for a different past; meet yourself where you are now.

- Do Mini-Workouts every day...yes, every single day. Make a conscious decision to enjoy it.

- Remember that consistency is the key, because it's the sum total that counts.

- Set realistic goals.

- Remember: repetition creates habits and habits are self-reinforcing.

- Celebrate the fact that you are able to walk and make a pact with yourself to walk every day. Walk everywhere you can.

- Live your life with mirth and laughter.

- Love and honor yourself every day because you deserve it.

If anyone scoffs and says that doing three of this or five of that or 10 of the other thing won't make any difference, you can acknowledge that no, *individually*, a few seconds or even a few minutes of movement won't do anything all by itself, but as part of a move-all-day routine, it will make a huge positive impact on your health and well-being because, like so many things in life...

It's the cumulative effect that matters!

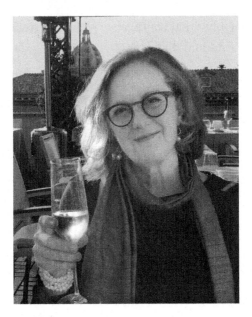

Here's to your success!

Dear Reader

If you're routinely doing Mini-Workouts and taking walks, I congratulate you! You have every reason to be proud of yourself for taking these important and meaningful steps toward a healthier and happier future.

For the time being, incorporating Mini-Workouts into your daily life and working your way up to walking two and a half hours a week may be all the change you can manage. I'm sure you know that in order to be truly healthy, nutritious foods should make up the majority of what's on your plate, but if the idea of making changes to your usual diet puts you in a panic, then give yourself time to adapt to your new style of more active living before tackling the eating part of the health equation. Remember, the idea is to be successful long term, not to feel guilty about what else you "should" or "should not" be doing.

When you're ready to move toward an even healthier future—and this means getting better control of what you're putting in your mouth—look for guidance that works for your personality type. It's important to avoid "miracle pills" and "instant-skinny" programs because they've never worked in the past and they won't work in the future; however, when you're ready to start enjoying nutritious food on a regular basis, there are many legitimate programs and resources to help, including a book by me (see my website for more info) that answers questions about diet, cooking, healthy options for entertaining, weight control, and general health, without jargon or false promises. Despite the steady recurrence of quick-fix claims, you can't lose weight "without dieting and exercise" unless you cut off a body part; you can't lose 100 pounds in 100 days and keep it off for good; and if there ever is a "magic diet pill" that really works, it will be front page news, not a "secret" that will only be revealed if you send a boatload of money to some unknown person or internet site. The only thing that will really get thinner from the latest fad by the modern version of a snake-oil salesman is your wallet. For now, let's just *get a move on!* and enjoy the abundant rewards that come from doing Mini-Workouts every day.

I wish you luck and I wish you well!

Acknowledgments

Just as a romaine leaf can't become a Caesar salad without cheese-makers, anchovy-catchers, lemon growers, and a cook, an idea can't become a book without the assistance of helpful professionals and the encouragement of friends. With that in mind, I give heartfelt thanks to the team at Bold Story Press: Founder and Publisher Emily Barrosse, who is giving voice and confidence to women writers; Karen Gulliver, who turned her gimlet eye upon my words and (tactfully) nudged them into order; Jeanne Schreiber, who knows how to turn a concept into eye-catching cover art and interior design; and the writing cohort who held me accountable. Thanks also to my dear friends and fellow word-nerds Sally Seymour and Mary Beth Glisson who read, proofread, and encouraged me along the way, and to Raffi, Hero, and Benny, the beloved rescues who keep my feet warm when I'm working and get me out walking every day, rain or shine or wildfires.

Of course, the most help has come from my best friend and life partner since bell-bottoms were in style, John Heymann, who cheerfully agreed that joining the

Peace Corps in our forties was a brilliant idea; who has led or followed me from the capitals of Europe to Ometepe Nicaragua to Oz to Jackson Hole to Machu Picchu and (repeatedly) to the beautiful beaches of Vieques Puerto Rico; who gets me and makes me laugh, and who has done the needful so I could write this book—thanks for the roller coaster ride.

And last, but by no means least, to my readers: thank you for believing that my hard-learned lessons can benefit you, too. I hope this book will help you on your journey to a healthier future and that you'll come to realize that you don't have to be perfect to be wonderful.

Luisa Coll-Pardo Heymann
Yountville, California

FOR MORE INFORMATION
OR TO CONTACT THE AUTHOR:

 HeymannLuisa@gmail.com

 Luisa.Heymann.Author

 HeymannLuisa

 luisaheymann

 Luisa Heymann

Bold Story Press is a curated, woman-owned hybrid publishing company with a mission of publishing well-written stories by women. If your book is chosen for publication, our team of expert editors and designers will work with you to publish a professionally edited and designed book. Every woman has a story to tell. If you have written yours and want to explore publishing with Bold Story Press, contact us at https://boldstorypress.com.

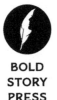

BOLD STORY PRESS

The Bold Story Press logo, designed by Grace Arsenault, was inspired by the nom de plume, or pen name, a sad necessity at one time for female authors who wanted to publish. The woman's face hidden in the quill is the profile of Virginia Woolf, who, in addition to being an early feminist writer, founded and ran her own publishing company, Hogarth Press.